O A C L
OXFORD AMERICAN CARDIOLOGY LIBRARY

Hypertension

O A C L
OXFORD AMERICAN CARDIOLOGY LIBRARY

Hypertension

George Bakris, MD, DMSc(Hon), FASH, FASN
Professor of Medicine
Director, Hypertension Center
University of Chicago Pritzker School of Medicine
Chicago, IL

Ragavendra R. Baliga, MD, MBA, FACP, FRCP (Edin), FACC
Editor-in-Chief, Heart Failure Clinics of North America
Associate Editor, Am Coll of Cardiology
    Cardiosource Journal Scan
Vice Chief & Asst Division Director
Division of Cardiovascular Medicine
Professor of Internal Medicine
The Ohio State University Medical Center
Columbus, OH

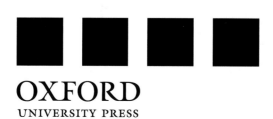

OXFORD
UNIVERSITY PRESS

OXFORD
UNIVERSITY PRESS

Oxford University Press is a department of the University of Oxford. It furthers the
University's objective of excellence in research, scholarship, and education by
publishing worldwide.

Oxford   New York
Auckland   Cape Town   Dar es Salaam   Hong Kong   Karachi
Kuala Lumpur   Madrid   Melbourne   Mexico City   Nairobi
New Delhi   Shanghai   Taipei   Toronto

With offices in
Argentina   Austria   Brazil   Chile   Czech Republic   France   Greece
Guatemala   Hungary   Italy   Japan   Poland   Portugal   Singapore
South Korea   Switzerland   Thailand   Turkey   Ukraine   Vietnam

Oxford is a registered trademark of Oxford University Press in the UK
and certain other countries.

Published in the United States of America by
Oxford University Press
198 Madison Avenue, New York, NY 10016

Library of Congress Cataloging-in-Publication Data

Hypertension / [edited by] George Bakris, Ragavendra R. Baliga.
   p. ; cm. — (Oxford American cardiology library)
Includes bibliographical references and index.
ISBN 978-0-19-975490-8 (pbk. : alk. paper)
I. Bakris, George L., 1952-   II. Baliga, R. R.   III. Series: Oxford American cardiology
library.
[DNLM: 1. Hypertension.   WG 340]
616.132—dc23   2011039915

9 8 7 6 5 4 3 2 1
Printed in the United States of America
on acid-free paper

Disclosures

Preface

More than 75 million Americans age 18 and older have hypertension and individuals who are normotensive at age 55 have a 90% lifetime risk for developing high blood pressure. Hypertension is the leading risk factor for stroke and cardiovascular disease. In individuals over the age of 50, systolic blood pressure is a more important than diastolic blood pressure as a risk factor for cardiovascular disease. Starting at 115/75 mm Hg, cardiovascular risk doubles with each increment of 20/10 mm Hg throughout the BP range. Therefore, those health-promoting lifestyle modifications help delay the development of cardiovascular disease and onset of hypertension. Reducing blood pressure can reduce stroke incidence by as much as 35–40%, the incidence of myocardial infarction by 20–25% and incidence of heart failure by 50%. With growing obesity epidemic hypertension prevalence will continue to grow as will diabetes. Together these diseases will be the leading causes of cardiovascular morbidity and mortality.

We invited an international group of experts to discuss and share their expertise regarding hypertension and its contribution to cardiovascular risk and updated opportunities to modify this risk. The authors are leaders in their field and share insights regarding new findings as they apply to clinical practice in their respective areas of research. We, therefore, hope that this book will serve as an informative and stimulating, up-to-date state-of-the art overview that will assist internists, primary care physicians, physician-extenders and specialists improve blood pressure control rates and reduce morbidity.

George Bakris, MD, DMSc(Hon), FASH, FASN
Professor of Medicine
Director, Hypertension Center
University of Chicago Pritzker School of Medicine
Chicago, IL

Ragavendra R. Baliga, MD, MBA, FACP (Edin), FACC,
Editor-in-Chief, Heart Failure Clinics of North America
Associate Editor, Am Coll of Cardiology
Cardiosource Journal Scan
Vice Chief & Asst Division Director
Division of Cardiovascular Medicine
Professor of Internal Medicine
The Ohio State University Medical Center
Columbus, OH

Contents

Contributors   *xi*

1 Impact of High Blood Pressure on Cardiovascular
   Risk and Benefits of Lowering Blood Pressure   1
2 Diagnosing Hypertension   15
3 Laboratory and Diagnostic Procedures   29
4 Treatment of Essential Hypertension   39

5 Managing Comorbidities
   a. Ischemic Heart Disease   55
   b. Heart Failure   59
   c. Diabetic Hypertension   65
   d. Chronic Kidney Disease   71
   e. Cerebrovascular Disease/Cognitive Function   83

6 Special Populations
   a. Hypertensive Urgencies and Emergencies   93
   b. Minorities   99
   c. Hypertension in Pregnancy   105
   d. Hypertension in Children and Adolescents   117
   e. Obesity and the Metabolic Syndrome   123
   f. Peripheral Arterial Disease   135

7 Improving Hypertension Control
   a. Adherence to Regimens   143
   b. Resistant Hypertension   151

8 Public Health Challenges and Community Programs   157

Appendix *163*

Index *167*

Contributors

Vasilios G. Athyros, MD

Head of the Atherosclerosis and
Metabolic Syndrome Units,
Second Propedeutic Department
of Internal Medicine
Medical School
Aristotle University of Thessaloniki
Hippokration Hospital
Thessaloniki, Greece

Shadi Barakat, MD

Division of Endocrinology,
Diabetes and Metabolism
University of Missouri
Harry S Truman VA Hospital
Columbia, MO

John D. Bisognano, MD, PhD

Professor of Medicine, Division of
Cardiology
Director of Cardiology Outpatient
Service
University of Rochester
Rochester, NY

Patrick Campbell, MD

Division of Hypertension and
Clinical Pharmacology
Pat and Jim Calhoun Cardiology
Center
University of Connecticut School
of Medicine
Farmington, CT

F. Gary Cunningham, MD

Professor and Beatrice and Miguel
Elias Distinguished Chair
Department of Obstetrics and
Gynecology
University of Texas Southwestern
Medical Center
Dallas, TX

Paula T. Einhorn, MD, MS

National Heart, Lung,
and Blood Institute
Bethesda, MD

William J. Elliott, MD, PhD

Professor of Preventive
Medicine, Internal Medicine and
Pharmacology
Head, Division of Pharmacology
The Pacific Northwest University
of Health Sciences
Yakima, WA

Bonita Falkner, MD

Professor of Medicine and
Pediatrics
Jefferson Medical College
Thomas Jefferson University
Philadelphia, PA

Sergio Chang Figueroa, MD

Division of Endocrinology,
Diabetes and Metabolism
University of Missouri
Harry S Truman VA Hospital
Columbia, MO

John M. Flack, MD, MPH

Professor and Chairman
Department of Internal
Medicine
Divisions of Endocrinology,
Metabolism, and Hypertension
and Translational Research
and Clinical Epidemiology, and
Department of Physiology
Wayne State University
Detroit Medical Center
Detroit, MI

CONTRIBUTORS

Philip B. Gorelick, MD, MPH
John S. Garvin Professor and Head
Director, Center for Stroke Research
Section of Stroke and Neurological
Critical Care
Department of Neurology and
Rehabilitation
University of Illinois College of
Medicine at Chicago
Chicago, IL

Clarence E. Grim, MS, MD
High Blood Pressure Consulting
Milwaukee, WI

Melissa Gunasekera, MD
University of Rochester Medical
Center
Rochester, NY

Asterios Karagiannis, MD
Professor of Internal Medicine
Second Propedeutic Department
of Internal Medicine
Medical School
Aristotle University of Thessaloniki
Hippokration Hospital
Thessaloniki, Greece

Michael R. Lattanzio, DO
Division of Nephrology
Department of Medicine
University of Maryland School of
Medicine
Baltimore, MD

Phillip Levy, MD, MPH
Associate Professor
Department of Emergency
Medicine
Wayne State University
Detroit, MI

**Marshall D. Lindheimer, MD,
FACP, FRCOG (London ad
eundem)**
Professor Emeritus
Departments of Obstetrics and
Gynecology and Medicine

The University of Chicago
Chicago, IL

**Donald M. Lloyd-Jones,
MD, ScM**
Chair, Department of Preventive
Medicine
Associate Professor in Preventive
Medicine and Medicine-Cardiology
Bluhm Cardiovascular Institute
Northwestern University Feinberg
School of Medicine
Chicago, IL

Amgad N. Makaryus, MD
Director of Echocardiography and
Cardiac CT and MRI
Department of Cardiology
North Shore University Hospital
Manhasset, NY

Victor Marinescu, MD, PhD
Department of Medicine
Divisions of Cardiology, Nutrition
and Preventive Medicine
William Beaumont Hospital
Royal Oak, MI

David Martins, MD, MS
Assistant Dean of Research and
Education
Program Director of the Clinical
Research Center
Charles Drew University of
Medicine and Science
Los Angeles, CA

**Peter A. McCullough,
MD, MPH**
Chief, Division of Nutrition and
Preventive Medicine
Division of Cardiology
Department of Medicine
William Beaumont Hospital
Royal Oak, MI

Samy I. McFarlane, MD, MPH
SUNY Downstate Medical Center
Brooklyn, NY

Dimitri P. Mikhailidis, MD

Academic Head of Department,
Reader & Honorary Consultant,
Department of Clinical Biochemistry
Royal Free Campus
University College London Medical
School
University College London
London, UK

William J. Mosley II, MD

Bluhm Cardiovascular Institute
Department of Medicine
Northwestern University Feinberg
School of Medicine
Chicago, IL

**Samar A. Nasser, PhD,
PAC, MPH**

Divisions of Endocrinology,
Metabolism and Hypertension and
Translational Research and Clinical
Epidemiology
Wayne State University
Detroit Medical Center
Detroit, MI

Keith Norris, MD

Executive Vice President for
Research and Health Affairs
Charles Drew University of
Medicine and Science
and
Professor of Medicine
Assistant Dean for Clinical and
Translational Sciences
David Geffen School of Medicine
at UCLA
Los Angeles, CA

Domenic A. Sica, MD

Professor of Medicine and
Pharmacology
Chairman, Clinical Pharmacology
and Hypertension
Virginia Commonwealth University
Health System
Richmond, VA

Manmeet M. Singh, MD

Assistant Professor
Department of Internal
Medicine
Division of General Internal
Medicine
Wayne State University
Detroit Medical Center
Detroit, MI

Matthew J. Sorrentino, MD

Professor of Medicine
Department of Medicine
Section of Cardiology
University of Chicago Pritzker
School of Medicine
Chicago, IL

James R. Sowers, MD

Professor of Medicine, Physiology
and Pharmacology
Director of Diabetes and
Cardiovascular Center
University of Missouri
Harry S Truman VA Hospital
Columbia, MO

**Fernando D. Testai,
MD, PhD**

Assistant Professor
of Neurology
Section of Stroke and Neurological
Critical Care
Department of Neurology and
Rehabilitation
University of Illinois College of
Medicine at Chicago
Chicago, IL

**Konstantinos Tziomalos,
MD, PhD**

First Propedeutic Department of
Internal Medicine
Medical School
Aristotle University
of Thessaloniki
AHEPA University Hospital
Thessaloniki, Greece

CONTRIBUTORS

Nosratola D. Vaziri, MD

Professor of Medicine, Physiology
and Biophysics
Chief, Division of Nephrology and
Hypertension, Medicine
University of California Irvine
School of Medicine
Irvine, CA

Matthew R. Weir, MD

Director, Division of Nephrology
Department of Medicine
University of Maryland Hospital,
Baltimore
and
Professor of Medicine
University of Maryland School of
Medicine
Baltimore, MD

Adam Whaley-Connell, MD

Assistant Professor of Medicine
Division of Nephrology
University of Missouri
Harry S Truman VA Hospital
Columbia, MO

William B. White, MD

Chief, Hypertension and Clinical
Pharmacology Division
Professor, Department of
Medicine
Division of Hypertension and
Clinical Pharmacology
Pat and Jim Calhoun Cardiology
Center
University of Connecticut School
of Medicine
Farmington, CT

**Gerda G. Zeeman,
MD, PhD**

Associate Professor, Department
of Obstetrics and Gynecology
University Medical Center
Groningen
Groningen, Netherlands

Chapter 1

Impact of High Blood Pressure on Cardiovascular Risk and Benefits of Lowering Blood Pressure

William J. Mosley II, MD, and
Donald M. Lloyd-Jones, MD, ScM

Introduction

Over the past century, we have come to recognize the substantial and causal role played by elevated blood pressure (BP) in increasing risk for cardiovascular disease (CVD). HTN is a major risk factor for CVD, the leading cause of death in American adults, treatment of which can reduce risk for CVD and extend life. The high prevalence of HTN, which affects 75 million American adults,[1] and its clear association with CVD make it a critical area of focus for public health and clinical initiatives.

There are several common measures that can be used to represent the level of BP: systolic BP (SBP) and diastolic BP (DBP), which represent the BP during their respective cardiac cycles; mean arterial pressure (MAP), the integrated mean of the pulsatile arterial pressure wave form (usually calculated as two thirds of the DBP plus one third of the SBP); mid-BP, the mean of SBP and DBP; and pulse pressure (PP), the difference between the SBP and DBP.[2] These different components are all associated with and predictive of incident cardiovascular events to varying degrees. In this chapter, we will discuss the age-related changes in BP, the detrimental impact of hypertension (HTN) on cardiovascular risk, the predictive value of various BP components on cardiovascular outcomes, and the benefits of lowering BP.

Age-Related Changes in BP

The hemodynamic patterns of BP across the age spectrum have been elegantly described by Franklin et al.[3] using data from the longstanding Framingham Heart

Study. Among participants ages 30 to 84 years, mean SBP tended to increase linearly with age, whereas DBP tended to increase up to age 50 years, plateau for 10 years, and then decline after 60 years of age. The divergence of SBP and DBP, particularly after age 50 years, causes a steep rise in PP, which tends to widen further after age 60 years. MAP tends to remain similar after age 50 to 60 years, since the DBP is falling and SBP is rising. In the younger population, younger than 50 years, isolated diastolic HTN is the most common type of HTN in untreated individuals (46.9%), whereas isolated systolic HTN becomes the most prevalent type by the fifth decade (54%), increasing to more than 87% by the sixth decade.[3]

Because most population studies have been limited to adults younger than 75 years, Lloyd Jones et al.[4] focused on the Framingham Heart Study elderly population (older than 80 years). They pooled data from more than 5,000 participants and grouped them according to BP stages (as defined by the Seventh Joint National Committee guidelines [JNC 7])[5] and ages less than 60, 60 to 79, and more than 80 years. As expected, the rising prevalence of HTN with age was confirmed starting at 27.3% in the youngest group and increasing to 63% in those 60 to 79 years and 74% in the oldest group. In addition, the prevalence of stage 2 HTN (SBP ≥160 mm Hg or DBP ≥100 mm Hg) increased with age, at 20%, 52%, and 60% in men aged less than 60, 60 to 79, and more than 80 years respectively; similar trends were observed in women.

Physiologically, the increase in BP with age can be explained by time- and risk factor-dependent fracturing and disarray of elastin in the vessel walls, replacement by collagen proliferation, and calcium deposits related to arteriosclerosis, all of which increase arterial stiffness of central capacitance vessels. This stiffening of the central arteries explains the rising SBP and PP and decreasing DBP after age 60. Stiff arteries have decreased elastic capacity and diminished elastic recoil of the capacitance arteries, causing a quicker runoff of stroke volume and lower central blood volume and pressure at the beginning of diastole. With the rise of SBP and fall of DBP, PP becomes a surrogate marker for increasing central arterial stiffness.[2]

Understanding Risk and Benefit

It is important to understand the terminology used to indicate the magnitude of harm associated with a risk factor like elevated BP, and the magnitude of benefit associated with its treatment. Absolute risk of disease associated with a given exposure is often expressed as the rate of development of new cases of disease per unit of time (or incidence) in exposed subjects. This proportion may be compared with the proportion among unexposed subjects in a variety of ways. The *relative risk* of disease is the ratio of disease incidence among exposed compared with non-exposed individuals. As such, relative risk measures the strength of the association between exposure and disease, but it gives no indication of the *absolute risk* of disease. For example, the relative risk for CVD associated with a given risk factor such as HTN might be three in a given population. This would be interpreted to mean that those with HTN have three times the chance of developing CVD as those without HTN. However, a relative risk of three might indicate substantial disease burden in one population and very little in another. If the rate of CVD in the non-hypertensive group is near zero, then three times that risk will still be a very low absolute rate of disease. However, if the rate of CVD in the non-hypertensive group is high (say, 10% over 5 years), then three times that rate may indicate a substantial amount of disease associated with HTN. To integrate the issues of relative risk, absolute risk, and prevalence of a risk factor, the *attributable risk* of a given exposure describes the amount of the incidence of disease in a population that can be ascribed to the exposure, assuming a causal relationship exists. The *population attributable risk* accounts for the proportion of individuals in the population who are exposed, as well as the relative risk. Therefore, attributable risk is a useful concept in determining the public health impact of a given risk factor and in selecting risk factors that should be targeted for prevention programs.

The benefit of a treatment in reducing risk for a given outcome may be described in several ways. When a treatment is compared with placebo (or with another treatment), the difference between the two groups may be described as an *absolute risk reduction* (the absolute difference in event rates between the two groups) or as a *relative risk reduction* (calculated as the difference between the two groups divided by the rate in the control group). As above, knowledge of the absolute risk difference is often more informative, and allows calculation of the *number-needed-to-treat* (calculated as [1/the absolute risk difference]), which represents the number of individuals who need to be treated to prevent one event in a given time frame. For example, if the result of a 5-year trial is that the event rate in the control group is 10% and the event rate in the treatment group is 5%, the relative risk reduction associated with treatment is 0.5 or 50% (0.10 − 0.05/0.10), the absolute risk reduction is 0.05 or 5% (0.10 − 0.05), and the number-needed-to-treat to prevent one event in 5 years is 20 (1/0.05). All of these measures should be considered in determining the efficacy of a proposed therapy.

Outcomes of Elevated BP

HTN is a well-established independent risk factor for the development of clinical CVD events. Higher BP level is associated with greater CVD risk in a continuous and graded fashion for all endpoints studied, including total mortality, CVD mortality, coronary heart disease (CHD) mortality, myocardial infarction (MI), heart failure (HF), left ventricular hypertrophy, atrial fibrillation, stroke/transient ischemic attack, peripheral vascular disease, and renal failure.[6–10] Individuals with untreated or treated HTN with BP at or above 140/90 mm Hg have a two- to three-fold increased risk for all CVD events combined, compared with normotensive individuals. Moreover, this risk is not limited to only those with HTN as defined by JNC 7.[5] Vasan et al.[9] demonstrated in a cohort of more than 6,000 men and women that, compared to those with optimal BP (<120/80 mm Hg), participants with high-normal BP (SBP 130 to 139 mm Hg or DBP 85 to 89 mm Hg) had a significant 1.6- to 2.5-fold increased adjusted risk for CVD. These findings have prompted a more aggressive approach to identify those with what are now called "prehypertensive" BP levels by the JNC 7 guideline.[5]

When considering the largest disease classes within CVD, the *relative* risks associated with HTN are greatest for stroke and HF, and lower for CHD. However, because the overall incidence of CHD in most populations is greater than that of stroke or HF, the absolute impact of HTN is more profound on CHD than other manifestations of CVD. It is therefore worth examining the individual associations of HTN with CHD, stroke, and HF.

HTN and CHD

BP is associated with a graded and continuous risk for CHD, which is the leading cause of death in American adults, responsible for 1 in 6 deaths per year.[1] Some of the most compelling data demonstrating the association between BP and CHD risk come from the Multiple Risk Factor Intervention Trial (MRFIT),[11,12] which assessed the incremental risk of elevated BP in more than 347,000 middle-aged men (35 to 57 years old) who were screened for enrollment. As shown in Figure 1.1A, there was a continuous and graded effect of BP on the multivariable-adjusted relative risk for CHD mortality beginning at pressures well below 140 mm Hg. The relative risk was clearly highest for men with SBP at or above 180 mm Hg; however, the vast majority of men at baseline had an SBP under 159 mm Hg. Thus, taking into account the number of men in each stratum and the expected rates of CHD death, a substantial number of excess CHD deaths occur at lower BP levels. Nearly two thirds of excess CHD deaths occurred in men with baseline SBP between 130 and 159 mm Hg (Fig. 1.1B), relatively "mild" levels of elevated BP.

The Prospective Studies Collaboration[7] showed that the association of BP level with elevated risk for CVD extended down even into the "optimal" range, defined as less than 120/80 mm Hg by current JNC guidelines.[5] This study, which was a large meta-analysis of 61 prospective observational studies including nearly 1 million individuals and 12.7 million person-years of follow-up of participants aged 40 to 89 years, examined the association of BP measures with several cardiovascular outcomes. The investigators found that at almost all ages, the risk for death from ischemic heart disease doubled for each increment of 20 mm Hg in SBP and 10 mm Hg in DBP, starting at a BP of 115/75 mm Hg. The risk in the oldest group, 80 to 89 years, increased by 50% in a similar fashion with escalating BP. Similarly, the Chicago Heart Association Detection Project in Industry, a study that included more than 10,000 men aged 18 to 39 years with 25 years of follow-up, found similar results. Multivariable-adjusted risk for CHD increased in a graded fashion for every increase of SBP by 15 mm Hg and DBP by 10 mm Hg starting at a reference of SBP 120 to 129 mm Hg and DBP of 70 to 79 mm Hg.[13] There was no significant difference in the reference group compared to those with BP less than 120/80 mm Hg. These collective studies

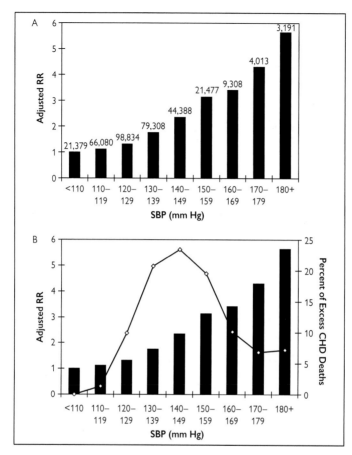

Figure 1.1 Relative risks for coronary heart disease (CHD) mortality among screenees for the Multiple Risk Factor Intervention Trial by level of systolic blood pressure (SBP; Panel A), with number of men in each stratum of SBP; and distribution of excess CHD deaths by SBP stratum (Panel B). (Data from Neaton JD, Kuller L, Stamler J, Wentworth DN. Impact of systolic and diastolic blood pressure on cardiovascular mortality. In: Laragh JH, Brenner BM, eds. Hypertension: Pathophysiology, Diagnosis, and Management, 2nd ed. Raven Press, 1995:127–144.)

emphasize the impact of HTN on CHD, but also highlight the inherent risk of prehypertension, which previously was thought to be benign.

HTN and Stroke

HTN is the dominant risk factor for both ischemic and hemorrhagic stroke—the third leading cause of death in the United States, after heart disease and cancer. There are more than 750,000 new or recurrent strokes per year, with more than 130,000 deaths per year attributed to stroke as the underlying cause.[1] The association of HTN with stroke persists even when considered in the context of other known risk factors, such as cigarette smoking, atrial fibrillation, MI, and diabetes. Those with a BP above 120/80 mm Hg compared to optimal BP have twice the lifetime risk of developing stroke.[14]

Similar to CHD, HTN is associated with a continuous graded risk for stroke that is not limited to frank HTN, but extends down into lower BP ranges. The Prospective Studies Collaboration,[7] in addition to ischemic heart disease, also evaluated stroke mortality outcomes across the spectrum of BP levels. For ages 40 to 79 years, the risk for stroke death more than doubled for each higher increment of 20 mm Hg in SBP and 10 mm Hg DBP, starting at a BP of 115/75 mm Hg.

HTN and HF

HF is reaching epidemic proportions as the prevalence of HTN increases, our population ages, and there is improved survival after MI. It is estimated that 5.8 million Americans have HF, which caused 1.1 million hospitalizations and was implicated in over 280,000 deaths in 2006. The burden of HF thus amounts to a large cost, projected to be $39.2 billion for 2010.[1]

Among individuals who develop HF, fully 75% have antecedent HTN. Similar to stroke, HTN is the dominant risk factor for HF. The overall remaining lifetime risk for HF is 1 in 5 for men and women age 40 and older, but at every age there is a stepwise increase in lifetime risk for HF with higher BP levels. The lifetime risk for those with BP at or above 160/90 mm Hg (stage 2 HTN) is double that of those with BP at or above 140/90 mm Hg.[15] Levy et al.[16] demonstrated the association of HTN with HF, observing hazard ratios of approximately two for men and three for women over the ensuing 18 years, compared to participants without HTN. These hazard ratios were far lower than the hazard ratios for HF associated with MI, which were greater than six for both men and women. However, the population prevalence of HTN was 60%, compared with approximately 6% for MI. Therefore, the population-attributable risk for HF from HTN (i.e., the fraction of HF in this population that could be eliminated if HTN were eradicated) was 59% in women and 39% in men. The population-attributable risk for MI was 13% for women and 34% for men.

Risk Factor Clustering

HTN infrequently occurs alone, and when present should alert the physician to look for other risk factors. HTN is an independent risk factor for CVD, but it confers even greater risk when the overall risk factor burden is considered. Data from Framingham, including a sample of more than 4,500 older individuals, revealed that among those with high-normal BP or HTN, only 2.4% had no other CVD risk factors, whereas 59.3% had at least one additional risk factor, and 38.2% already had target organ damage, clinical CVD or diabetes (Fig. 1.2).[17] Moreover, when HTN is added to multivariable prediction models along with

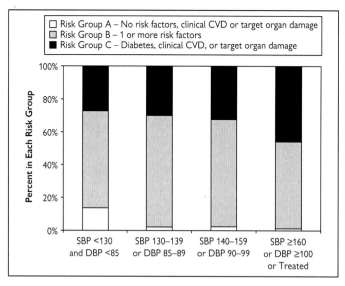

Figure 1.2 Cross-classification of risk groups and BP stages among 4,962 Framingham Heart Study subjects. (Data from Lloyd-Jones DM, Evans JC, Larson MG, O'Donnell CJ, Wilson PW, Levy D. Cross-classification of JNC VI blood pressure stages and risk groups in the Framingham Heart Study. Arch Intern Med 1999;159(18):2206–2212.)

other risk factors, the risk for CHD increases substantially, and it increases even more in the presence of greater burden of other risk factors (Fig. 1.3).

Predictive Utility of BP Measures

Over the past several decades, there has been considerable debate about which BP measure is the best marker of risk for CVD outcomes. In the 1950s, severe diastolic HTN was initially the focus of treatment because of the associated increased mortality in the young, in whom diastolic HTN is most prevalent. In addition, systolic HTN was thought to be part of the natural aging process, and HTN in general had limited effective treatments. In the late 1960s, the VA Cooperative trial demonstrated that treatment of diastolic HTN reduced risks for stroke and HF, which spurred the creation of the National High Blood Pressure Education Program (NHBPEP) and eventually the first Report of the Joint National Committee on Detection, Evaluation, and Treatment of High BP (JNC) in 1976. These first guidelines focused on DBP. Over time, research has demonstrated the greater predictive value of SBP in individuals older than 50 years, thus changing the emphasis in the guidelines from DBP to SBP, culminating in the recommendations of JNC 7.[5]

The totality of current evidence supports SBP as the easiest and best predictor for CVD over DBP and PP. Mid-BP and MAP have also been evaluated

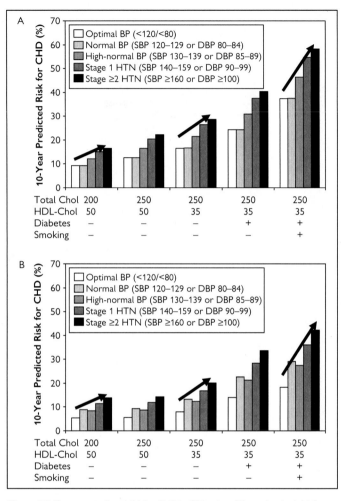

Figure 1.3 Ten-year predicted risk for CHD by BP level at different levels of risk factor burden for a man (Panel A) and a woman (Panel B) at age 60 years.

in a limited number of studies, with evidence suggesting even greater predictive value over SBP and DBP, but these measurements are less practical to perform on a regular basis.[2] The dominance of SBP was first recognized by Kannel et al.[18] but was not generally accepted until decades later. In addition to determining the continuous graded effect of BP on CHD, MRFIT investigators also reported the greater predictive value of SBP as compared to DBP.[11] Men greater than 50 years old with isolated systolic HTN (SBP >160, DBP <90 mm Hg) had the highest 12-year CHD and mortality rates compared to those with diastolic

HTN and normotension. When all participants were stratified into quintiles of SBP or DBP, risks for each SBP quintile were the same or higher than for the corresponding quintile of DBP. Moreover, when stratified by JNC BP stages of SBP and DBP, SBP was associated with greater risk for CHD mortality than DBP in each JNC BP stage.[12]

The MRFIT data have been corroborated by more recent studies highlighting SBP as a more robust marker for the spectrum of CVD events, including CHD, HF, and stroke. Investigators from the Cardiovascular Health Study of older Americans noted that every 1-standard-deviation increment in SBP was associated with higher adjusted risk for CHD and stroke than a 1-standard-deviation increment in DBP (Fig. 1.4).[19] The Chicago Heart Association Detection Project in Industry investigators, who evaluated a large cohort of more than 30,000 men and women free of CVD at baseline over 33 years of follow-up, also demonstrated that SBP was a superior predictor of CHD, HF, and stroke outcomes, in terms of relative and absolute risks and measures of model fit and discrimination.[20]

In recent literature, PP has been shown to be associated significantly with incident CHD, HF, and stroke. Specifically, when DBP is considered in the context of the SBP level, an inverse association for DBP and CHD risk has been observed, illustrating the association of PP with CVD.[2,18,19] The Chicago Heart Association Detection Project in Industry studied the association of PP with CHD, HF, and stroke outcomes. Consistent with some of the prior literature, this large study with extended follow-up showed that PP was a weaker

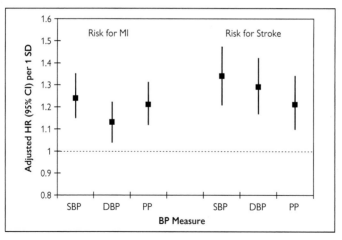

Figure 1.4 Adjusted hazard ratios (95% confidence intervals) for MI and stroke per each 1 standard deviation (SD) increment in SBP (SD = 21.4 mm Hg), DBP (SD = 11.2 mm Hg), and PP (SD = 18.5 mm Hg). (Data from Psaty BM, Furberg CD, Kuller LH, et al. Association between blood pressure level and the risk of myocardial infarction, stroke, and total mortality: the Cardiovascular Health Study. Arch Intern Med 2001;161(9):1183–1192.)

predictor of CVD events than SBP. Moreover, Bayes' information criteria values and areas under receiver-operating characteristic curves all indicated better predictive utility for SBP and DBP compared with PP.[20] The major limitation of PP is that it incorporates information from two BP components (SBP and DBP) and is a "floating" variable. It has no relation to an absolute BP level: for example, a PP of 60 mm Hg could be associated with BP of 180/120 mm Hg or 120/60 mm Hg.

In conclusion, higher BP levels, starting within the range currently considered optimal, are associated with increased risk for all manifestations of CVD, including CHD, stroke, and HF. This burden becomes more pronounced when additional risk factors such as age, sex, smoking, cholesterol level, and diabetes are considered in addition to HTN. And, indeed, individuals with elevated BP almost invariably have other risk factors present, increasing their risks. We have also learned that SBP is the most robust and practical way for assessing BP and predicting outcomes. As reviewed in the next section, treating and lowering BP can markedly decrease the risk and impact of BP on CVD and mortality.

Impact of Treatment of HTN

Although the goals of HTN treatment have changed over the past 50 years, it is well established that treatment of elevated BP reduces the incidence of CVD. As discussed previously, DBP was initially the BP component of concern given the premature death seen in the young with diastolic HTN. The first trial to show benefit in treatment of HTN was the VA Cooperative Trial.[21] In this trial 143 men, with a mean age of 51 years and DBP levels averaging between 115 and 129 mm Hg, were followed for 16 to 21 months. They were randomized to active antihypertensive treatment versus placebo. The treatment group had a significant decline in DBP by an average of 30 mm Hg, whereas the placebo group had no significant change. A significant reduction in severe cardiovascular events—death, stroke, HF, and MI—was observed with active treatment (N = 2) versus placebo (N = 27). This trial was followed with a larger VA Cooperative trial over 5 years that evaluated a similar population with less severe diastolic HTN, averaging 90 to 114 mm Hg. In this trial, active treatment also produced a significant reduction in cardiovascular events in the treatment group, with more than a 30% relative reduction in events compared with placebo.[20] As previously mentioned, these trials collectively spurred the creation of the JNC guidelines in 1976, which initially focused on DBP as the main treatment goal.

Several trials and meta-analyses in the past several decades have shown the benefit of lowering both SBP and DBP.[21–25] Using network meta-analysis, a technique that combines direct and indirect evidence, cardiovascular outcomes were evaluated with various first-line antihypertensives in 42 long-term randomized placebo and active treatment controlled trials. This study[22] included numerous landmark trials that randomized a total of 192,478 patients with uncontrolled HTN who were free of HF and without a history of MI to seven major treatment strategies, including placebo. Overall, when all treatment strategies were collectively pooled, active treatment, compared to placebo, no treatment, or usual care, was associated with significant reductions in event rates by 10% to 46% in CHD, stroke, HF, CVD mortality, and total mortality. Of the first-line treatment strategies, low-dose diuretics were superior to all other treatments, including beta-blockers, angiotensin-converting enzyme inhibitors (ACE-Is), calcium channel blockers (CCBs), alpha-blockers, and angiotensin receptor blockers (ARBs). Compared with placebo, low-dose diuretics showed a significant reduction in CHD (relative risk [RR] 0.79; 95% confidence interval [CI], 0.69–0.92), HF (RR 0.51; 95% CI, 0.42–0.62), stroke (RR 0.71; 95% CI 0.63–0.81), composite CVD events (RR 0.76; 95% CI, 0.69–0.83), CVD mortality (RR 0.81; 95% CI, 0.73–0.92), and total mortality (RR 0.90; 95% CI, 0.84–0.96). Compared with other active treatments, low-dose diuretics were associated with a further relative risk reduction for CVD of 11% compared with beta-blockers, 6% compared with CCBs or ACE-Is, and 16% compared with alpha-blockers. It is important to mention that this analysis preserved within-trial comparisons of treatment strategies without any adjustment for in-trial BP differences. The BPs in low-dose diuretic trials were on average 3 to 5 mm Hg lower than other treatment strategies. Although this is a small difference, this may account for the demonstrated advantage of low-dose diuretic therapy.[22]

A more recent meta-analysis of 154 randomized trials of 464,000 subjects also examined antihypertensive treatments in the prevention of CVD while accounting for BP differences between treatment strategies, but also included patients with previous CVD.[23] This study sought to answer lingering uncertainty about the efficacy of different classes of antihypertensive agents. The subjects were separated into three groups: those with no history of vascular disease, a history of CHD, and a history of stroke. As seen in the previous meta-analysis, BP reduction by antihypertensive medication (thiazides, beta-blockers, ACE-Is, ARBs, CCBs) were effective in reducing cardiovascular events in all three groups by 15% to 36%. When BP levels were accounted for, certain antihypertensives were more effective in treating and preventing CVD. In patients with CHD, beta-blockers had a greater RR reduction of 29% compared to other treatments (15%); however, this benefit was limited to those with a recent MI. The other drug classes showed a similar reduction in CHD associated with BP reduction. All drugs also showed similar reductions in stroke, with the exception of CCBs, which were associated with a 9% greater RR of stroke. With regard to RR for HF, all classes were similar except CCBs, which were not as effective, having 5% less of a RR reduction.

SBP as Goal of Treatment

The current JNC 7 guidelines focus on SBP as the main indicator of need for treatment and the target for achieving control for the vast majority of patients with HTN. The superiority of SBP as a risk marker for CVD has been demonstrated, as has the reduction of CVD with treatment of BP targeting SBP. A meta-analysis of 10 trials[26] specifically addressed the question of whether, after treatment of SBP, there was benefit in lowering of DBP. The trials included were those evaluating active antihypertensive treatment versus placebo or no treatment in the young (N = 12,903, ages 30 to 49), the old (N = 14,329, ages 60 to 79), and the very old (N = 1209, age ≥80). BP was reduced by 8.3 to 10.7 mm Hg systolic and 3.2 to 4.6 mm Hg diastolic. Antihypertensive treatment reduced CVD events, stroke, and MI in all age groups to a similar extent. Lowering of DBP was not associated with a further reduction in CVD events as long as SBP was substantially decreased (defined as a decrease greater than the median reduction of 18 to 30 mm Hg). The average starting BP in the trials included was 166 to 177/85 to 88 mm Hg. This study supported other trials in demonstrating the effect of antihypertensive therapy, but also showed that when SBP is treated to within the goal range of current JNC guidelines (SBP <140 mm Hg), this may be an acceptable treatment goal without need for focus on DBP.[26]

Treatment in the Elderly

Treatment of HTN in the oldest old (>80 years of age) was also recently shown to be of benefit for reducing CVD events and total mortality in the later stages of life. Until the HYVET trial we only had limited data with small numbers focusing on this population, which led to apprehension in physicians treating this population. Previous studies showed a reduction in CVD events by up to 39%, but a CVD mortality benefit was not shown and there was concern for an increase in all-cause mortality.[8] The HYVET[27] trial, a randomized prospective trial of 3,845 men and women, evaluated patients over 80 years old. Participants were randomized to a thiazide diuretic (indapamide) or placebo therapy and followed up for 2 years. An ACE-I (or matching placebo) was added if necessary to achieve goal BP of less than 150/80 mm Hg. Active treatment was associated with a significant RR reduction in fatal and non-fatal stroke by 30%, and a 39% reduction in stroke death. CVD deaths were reduced by 23%, and all-cause mortality was also significantly reduced by 21%. The number-needed-to-treat with active therapy to prevent one death was 40 patients over 2 years. This trial demonstrated the safety and efficacy of antihypertensive treatment in the oldest old.

Conclusion

HTN is a major, causal contributor to the overwhelming prevalence and incidence of CVD in the United States. Elevations in BP, starting even in the "normal" ranges defined by JNC guidelines, is associated with increased risk of CVD, including stroke, HF, and CHD. Moreover, elevated BP increases risk even further when other risk factors for CVD are present, as they invariably are. For the present, CVD risk is best predicted using SBP levels for the vast majority of patients. Although HTN can result in highly morbid conditions and death, CVD events and mortality can be substantially reduced with a variety of effective antihypertensive agents in all age groups.

References

1. Lloyd-Jones D, Adams RJ, Brown TM, Carnethon M, Dai S, De Simone G, et al. Heart Disease and Stroke Statistics—2010 Update. *Circulation* 2010; 121(7):e46–e215.

2. Mosley WJ, 2nd, Greenland P, Garside DB, Lloyd-Jones DM. Predictive utility of pulse pressure and other blood pressure measures for cardiovascular outcomes. *Hypertension* 2007;49(6):1256–1264.

3. Franklin SS, Gustin WT, Wong ND, Larson MG, Weber MA, Kannel WB, et al. Hemodynamic patterns of age-related changes in blood pressure. The Framingham Heart Study. *Circulation* 1997;96(1):308–315.

4. Lloyd-Jones DM, Evans JC, Larson MG, O'Donnell CJ, Levy D. Differential impact of systolic and diastolic blood pressure level on JNC-VI staging. *Hypertension* 1999;34(3):381–385.

5. Chobanian AV, Bakris GL, Black HR, Cushman WC, Green LA, Izzo JL, Jr, et al. Seventh Report of the Joint National Committee on Prevention, Detection, Evaluation, and Treatment of High Blood Pressure. *Hypertension*. 2003;42(6):1206–1252.

6. Kannel WB, Wilson PWF. Cardiovascular risk factors and hypertension. In: Izzo JL, Jr., Black HR, eds. *Hypertension Primer: The Essentials of High Blood Pressure Basic Science, Population Science, and Clinical Management*, 4th ed. Philadelphia: Lippincott Williams & Wilkins, 2008:244–248.

7. Lewington S, Clarke R, Qizilbash N, Peto R, Collins R. Age-specific relevance of usual blood pressure to vascular mortality: a meta-analysis of individual data for one million adults in 61 prospective studies. *Lancet*. 2002;360(9349):1903–1913.

8. Mosley WJ, 2nd, Lloyd-Jones DM. Epidemiology of hypertension in the elderly. *Clin Geriatr Med* 2009;25(2):179–189.

9. Vasan RS, Larson MG, Leip EP, Evans JC, O'Donnell CJ, Kannel WB, et al. Impact of high-normal blood pressure on the risk of cardiovascular disease. *N Engl J Med* 2001;345(18):1291–1297.

10. Lloyd-Jones D, Levy D. Epidemiology of hypertension. In: Black HR, Elliott WJ, eds. *Hypertension: A Companion to Braunwald's Heart Disease*, 1st ed. Philadelphia: Saunders, 2007.

11. Rutan GH, Kuller LH, Neaton JD, Wentworth DN, McDonald RH, Smith WM. Mortality associated with diastolic hypertension and isolated systolic hypertension among men screened for the Multiple Risk Factor Intervention Trial. *Circulation* 1988;77(3):504–514.

12. Neaton JD, Kuller L, Stamler J, Wentworth DN. Impact of systolic and diastolic blood pressure on cardiovascular mortality. In: Laragh JH, Brenner BM, eds. *Hypertension: Pathophysiology, Diagnosis, and Management*, 2nd ed. New York: Raven Press, 1995:127–144.

13. Miura K, Daviglus ML, Dyer AR, Liu K, Garside DB, Stamler J, et al. Relationship of blood pressure to 25-year mortality due to coronary heart disease, cardiovascular diseases, and all causes in young adult men: the Chicago Heart Association Detection Project in Industry. *Arch Intern Med* 2001;161(12):1501–1508.

14. Seshadri S, Beiser A, Kelly-Hayes M, Kase CS, Au R, Kannel WB, et al. The lifetime risk of stroke: Estimates from the Framingham Study. *Stroke* 2006;37(2):345–350.

15. Lloyd-Jones DM, Larson MG, Leip EP, Beiser A, D'Agostino RB, Kannel WB, et al. Lifetime risk for developing congestive heart failure: the Framingham Heart Study. *Circulation.* 2002;106(24):3068–3072.

16. Levy D, Larson MG, Vasan RS, Kannel WB, Ho KK. The progression from hypertension to congestive heart failure. *JAMA* 1996;275(20):1557–1562.

17. Lloyd-Jones DM, Evans JC, Larson MG, O'Donnell CJ, Wilson PW, Levy D. Cross-classification of JNC VI blood pressure stages and risk groups in the Framingham Heart Study. *Arch Intern Med* 1999;159(18):2206–2212.

18. Dustan HP. 50th anniversary historical article. Hypertension. *J Am Coll Cardiol* 1999;33(3):595–597.

19. Psaty BM, Furberg CD, Kuller LH, Cushman M, Savage PJ, Levine D, et al. Association between blood pressure level and the risk of myocardial infarction, stroke, and total mortality: the cardiovascular health study. *Arch Intern Med* 2001;161(9):1183–1192.

20. Mosley WJ, Greenland P, Garside DB, Lloyd-Jones DM. Predictive utility of pulse pressure and other blood pressure measures for cardiovascular outcomes. *Hypertension* 2007;49:1256–1264.

21. Effects of treatment on morbidity in hypertension. Results in patients with diastolic blood pressures averaging 115 through 129 mm Hg. *JAMA* 1967;202(11):1028–1034.

22. Effects of treatment on morbidity in hypertension. II. Results in patients with diastolic blood pressure averaging 90 through 114 mm Hg. *JAMA* 1970;213(7):1143–1152.

23. Law MR, Morris JK, Wald NJ. Use of blood pressure lowering drugs in the prevention of cardiovascular disease: meta-analysis of 147 randomised trials in the context of expectations from prospective epidemiological studies. *BMJ* 2009;338:1665.

24. Psaty BM, Lumley T, Furberg CD, Schellenbaum G, Pahor M, Alderman MH, et al. Health outcomes associated with various antihypertensive therapies used as first-line agents: a network meta-analysis. *JAMA* 2003;289(19):2534–2544.

25. Wang JG, Staessen JA, Franklin SS, Fagard R, Gueyffier F. Systolic and diastolic blood pressure lowering as determinants of cardiovascular outcome. *Hypertension* 2005;45(5):907–913.

26. JG, Staessen JA, Franklin SS, Fagard R, Gueyffier F. Systolic and diastolic blood pressure lowering as determinants of cardiovascular outcome. *Hypertension* 2005;45(5):907–913.

27. Beckett NS, Peters R, Fletcher AE, Staessen JA, Liu L, Dumitrascu D, et al. Treatment of hypertension in patients 80 years of age or older. *N Engl J Med* 2008;358(18):1887–1898.

Chapter 2

Diagnosing Hypertension

Patrick Campbell, MD, and William B. White, MD

HTN affects more than 75 million people in the United States, many of whom are not even aware they have the disease. In addition, the prevalence of HTN is on the rise as a result of the growing obesity epidemic. Consensus reports state that the lifetime risk of developing HTN is approximately 85% in the general population.[1] The cardiovascular (CV) risk that results from HTN is progressive with increasing BP levels. For every 20-mm Hg increase in SBP and every 10 mm Hg in DBP there is a doubling of the risk of death from CV diseases.[2] Furthermore, the accumulated data from multiple clinical trials have confirmed that even small increases in BP (3 to 5 mm Hg) are associated with substantial increases in CV risk. Obviously, the risk associated with HTN cannot be modified unless identified, and data from NHANES[3] indicate that approximately 30% of Americans are unaware of their elevated BP, and that approximately 50% of those aware that they have HTN have achieved their BP goal.[4] The importance of this lack of awareness and moderate rates of control is highlighted by a recent study that demonstrated that both untreated and uncontrolled patients with HTN have significantly higher all-cause and cardiovascular mortality than the general population.[5]

During the initial evaluation process for a patient who has HTN, the goals include:

1. To determine if the BP elevation is sustained
2. To evaluate and assess all CV risk factors
3. To assess for evidence of target organ damage
4. To identify potential secondary and/or reversible causes of HTN

BP Measurement

BP measurement has traditionally been performed in the clinician's office; however, with improved and validated technology and programmatic patient education, BPs can now be accurately assessed outside of the office setting. Although controversy exists over the most effective means of assessment (each modality has its own benefits and limitations), all three major methods described below can be used to complement each other and provide information to improve clinical decision-making.

Office BP Measurements

Benefits and Limitations

The traditional office BP measurement is the most common method used for the diagnosis and management of HTN. Office BPs measured by the physician or nurse that are standardized are useful since they are easily and rapidly interpretable as the measurement used in clinical trials and evidence-based guideline development. However, the utility of the office BP can be offset by several limitations, including high levels of variability, potential observer biases, as well as the "white coat effect." In the current hustle and bustle of a modern medical practice, the measurement of office BP may actually lose a significant amount of accuracy because of rushed measurements, improper technique and incorrect cuff size, the use of a single measurement, terminal digit preference, and digit preference/bias.[6-10]

Terminal digit bias is the practice of rounding the terminal digit to a particular number—typically zero—and can result in misdiagnoses and improper evaluation of medication efficacy. Terminal digit bias occurs in 30% to 40% of BP readings taken even in a specialist's practice.[6] Terminal digit bias results in either over- or underestimation of BP and can have an important clinical effect on disease management. It has been estimated that for each 10% increase in terminal digit bias there is an 8% reduction in the likelihood of a patient receiving appropriate antihypertensive therapy.[7]

Digit preference is caused by the bias of the observer taking the measurement, previous patient readings, or preset cutoffs or cuff inflation. These examples highlight the importance of education, proper training, and close monitoring to ensure accurate BP measurements in the clinical practice.

Measurement Technique

Issues concerning proper BP measurement technique include patient position, cuff size, cuff placement, stethoscope placement, and rates of deflation during auscultation. During measurements, patients should preferably be seated on a chair with their back supported, legs uncrossed, and arm supported at the level of the right atrium (mid-sternum). Ideally, the patient should be given 5 minutes to relax in the exam room and should be instructed not to talk during the readings. To reduce the impact of the pressor response to the observer and the environment, an average of three to five readings should be obtained, discarding the first reading. Appropriate cuff and bladder size is of utmost importance, as a small bladder size will overestimate the BP.[8] The cuff and bladder should encompass at least 80% of the arm circumference and should be 40% of the arm width. The American Heart Association has developed recommendations for cuff size based on arm circumference (Table 2.1). During the initial visit BP should be measured in both arms, and if the patient is on antihypertensive therapy or is over 65 years of age orthostatic measurements are recommended. The practitioner must pay close attention to the placement of the cuff and the stethoscope. The proper rate of inflation and deflation (approximately 2 to 3 mm Hg/second) should be followed to avoid

Table 2.1 Recommended Cuff/Bladder Size		
Arm Circumference (cm)	Cuff bladder Size (cm)	Standard Nomenclature
22–26	12 × 22	Small Adult
27–34	16 × 30	Adult
35–44	16 × 36	Large Adult
45–52	16 × 42	Adult Thigh

Reprinted with permission from Pickering TG, Hall JE, Appel LJ, et al. Recommendations for blood pressure measurement in humans and experimental animals: Part 1: Blood pressure measurement in humans: A statement for professionals from the Subcommittee of Professional and Public Education of the American Heart Association Council on High Blood Pressure Research. *Circulation* 2005;111:697–716.

inaccurate readings. Inflating the cuff to a pressure that ablates the radial pulse and using slow deflation rates will also help to avoid missing an auscultatory gap, which typically occurs in older patients with a wide pulse pressure. The initial Korotkoff sounds disappear between the SBP and DBP, only to reappear as the cuff is deflated. The presence of the auscultatory gap is a result of arteriosclerosis that leads to changes in the physical properties of the artery that prevent the vascular wall from resonating on opening. Additionally, during cuff deflation, underdeveloped Korotkoff sounds may make it impossible to auscultate the sounds when the compressed segment of the artery opens, disallowing the proximal and distal portions of the artery to communicate. In hypertensive patients the presence of the auscultatory gap is associated with increased CV risk.[11] Furthermore, missing the auscultatory gap can result in underestimation of the SBP.

In addition to the measurement issues noted above, multiple patient and environmental factors can affect the accuracy of office BP measurements. Recent ingestion of caffeinated beverages, exam rooms in which the ambient temperature is below room temperature, muscle tension or stress, pain, a full bladder, anxiety, very recent smoking, talking, and the white coat effect can all affect the precision of BP measurements. It is advisable for patients to avoid caffeine and nicotine for at least 60 minutes before their visit and to empty their bladder prior to the BP measurements.

Devices

Use of automated or semi-automated digital BP devices may have the potential to reduce some of the biases associated with manual (aneroid or mercury column) BP measurements. Automated oscillometric devices allow for multiple readings, decrease observer and digit bias, reduce the white coat effect, and correlate more accurately with 24-hour ambulatory BPs.[12–14] Prior to use of digital BP devices, it is strongly recommended that the device undergo a standard, independent clinical validation according to the guidelines of the Association of Advancement of Medical Instrumentation (AAMI) or the British Hypertension Society (BHS). A list of validated automated devices can be found at www.dableducational.com.

Special Clinical Situations that May Lead to Measurement Error

The white coat effect (or isolated office HTN) is generally defined when the office BP is above 140/90 mm Hg but ambulatory BP values are 130/80 mm Hg or less. This diagnosis has been reported to occur in as many as 20% to 35% of patients diagnosed with HTN.[15] Until recently white coat HTN was considered a benign phenomenon; recent studies with more than 10 years of follow-up show a transition of CV risk in patients with white coat HTN compared with normotensive patients.[16] However, it is unknown whether white coat HTN predicts the development of sustained HTN or there is another mechanism of increased CV risk, so these patients should be followed closely for the development of target organ damage and/or progression to sustained HTN.

Home Blood Pressure Measurements

Benefits and Limitations

Home (or self) BP measurements can add a great deal of information to the conventional office BP measurements. They allow multiple out-of-office readings that can aid in the management of the hypertensive patient. Home BP monitoring is also relatively inexpensive and has been shown to improve patient compliance with antihypertensive drug regimens.[17] Still, there are a number of limitations of home BP monitoring, including reporting bias by patients: as many as 50% of patients omit or fabricate self-recorded BP readings.[18]

Guidelines have suggested that optimal home BP values should be lower than office BP readings (Table 2.2). Home BP measurements have been shown to correlate more closely with CV outcomes (CV mortality, stroke) and target organ damage (left ventricular hypertrophy, proteinuria) than office BP measurements.[17–19]

Technique

Similar to office BP measurements, proper technique and patient position are important for self-BP measurements. Patients should wait to initiate BP measurements after they have been at rest for 3 to 5 minutes and should have an empty bladder and avoid eating, exercise, caffeine, or nicotine for 30 to 60 minutes prior to recording the pressure. All readings should be taken on the upper

Table 2.2 Normal BP Reading Based on Method of Measurement			
Method of Measurement	Optimal Blood Pressure (mm Hg)	Normal Blood Pressure (mm Hg)	Hypertensive (mm Hg)
Office	≤130/80	≤135/85	≥140/90
Home/Self	≤125/76	≤130/80	≥135/85
Ambulatory	≤125/75	≤130/80	≥130/80
24-hr average	≤130/80	≤135/85	≥135/85
Awake average	≤115/65	≤120/75	
Sleep average			

arm (brachial artery) with the arm supported at the level of the heart. Three readings should be taken in succession, separated by 1 minute, and averaged. Current consensus guidelines recommend duplicate premedication measurement in the morning and evening for 7 days performed every 3 months as a means to assess HTN control in treated patients.[19,20]

Devices

Selection of an appropriate device is essential to obtaining accurate home BP readings. While the number of commercially available devices has increased dramatically over the past decade, very few devices have been adequately validated. Both the BHS[21] and AAMI[22] have developed validation protocols for home BP devices, but unfortunately the vast majority of devices available on the market have not undergone such independent testing. The American Society of Hypertension recommends use of only validated home BP devices that are designed for use on the upper arm.[18] Wrist and finger devices are less accurate and are highly sensitive to changes in arm position. A complete and updated list of validated devices can be found at www.dableducational.com or www.bhsoc.org.

Special Clinical Situations

Consensus groups have advocated self-BP measurements as a means of screening for the diagnosis of both masked and white coat HTN. Masked HTN is a clinical condition in which the BP levels recorded in the office are substantially lower than those that occur at home and ambulatory BP values. The prevalence of masked HTN is unknown in the general population but is estimated to be 10% to 20% in the hypertensive population.[23] The Self-Measurement of Blood Pressure at Home in the Elderly: Assessment and Follow-up (SHEAF) study has shown that patients with masked HTN have CV risk profiles similar to that of sustained hypertensive patients.[24]

White coat HTN, essentially the opposite BP pattern of masked HTN, is the presence of isolated elevated office BP and normotension at home and on ambulatory monitoring. Home BP monitoring has been shown to have an intermediate sensitivity and high specificity (65% and 85% respectively)[25,26] for the detection of white coat HTN. Consensus reports have advocated that home BP monitoring should be used as a primary screening tool for the evaluation of white coat HTN.[27]

Ambulatory Blood Pressure Measurement

Benefits and Limitations

Originally reserved for CV research departments, the clinical usefulness of ambulatory BP monitoring has greatly expanded. Improved technology, noninvasive measurements, and prognostic data transformed ambulatory BP monitoring from a research tool to a clinical test. Numerous studies have shown that mean ambulatory BPs are lower than mean clinic BPs and correlate better with hypertensive target organ damage.[27–29]

Ambulatory BP measurements have shown stronger associations with prognosis for CV morbidity and mortality than office BP.[29,30] Additionally, ambulatory BP measurement has many advantages over office BP, including superior reproducibility, more accurate diagnosis of white coat HTN, the ability to evaluate nocturnal patterns of BP, diagnosis of masked HTN, assessment of early-morning BP surge, and improved determination of therapy efficacy (Fig. 2.1). It is generally agreed that the 24-hour BP should be lower than office BP due to the impact of sleep on BP. Values in Table 2.2 show the current expert opinion on comparable office and ambulatory pressures. Limitations of ambulatory BP monitoring include a high cost of equipment, software, and technical assistance, difficulty in monitoring in patients with chronic arrhythmias such as atrial fibrillation, and practical issues associated with monitoring in patients with very large arm circumferences (>42 to 45 cm mid-arm).

Technique

In most circumstances, the ABP device should be placed with an appropriate cuff size on the nondominant arm to avoid limitations in activities during work and awake periods. Patients should be instructed to perform their daily activities as usual but avoid strenuous exercise or heavy lifting. Interference with oscillometric algorithms is also problematic if patients spend long periods of time driving a vehicle. During cuff deflation, it is advisable for patients to keep the arm still to avoid motion artifact. Most ambulatory BP monitoring protocols call for recording the BP at 15-minute intervals while the patient is awake and at 20- to 30-minute intervals during sleep. It is important that more than 80% of the programmed measurements are obtained to provide appropriate quality for a 24-hour mean. Many ambulatory BP equipment manufacturers have developed software that provides descriptive statistics of the data, including means of the entire study period, the daytime/awake and nighttime/sleep BPs and heart rates, as well as proportional changes between daytime and nighttime.

Devices

It is only appropriate to use independently validated ambulatory recorders according to the guidelines of AAMI and BHS. The www.dableducational.com and www.bhsoc.org websites provide a list of updated and validated monitors. In addition to providing information on the accuracy of the ambulatory BP devices versus a standard, information on the reliability of the device and ease of use is often available in validation studies of these devices as well.

Special Clinical Situations

Ambulatory BP monitoring obtains an accurate 24-hour BP profile of patients during the normal activities of daily living. While these measurements were used initially to rule out important white coat effects, use of the technology is much broader and includes the assessment of masked HTN in treated or untreated individuals, assessment for symptomatic HTN and hypotension, and

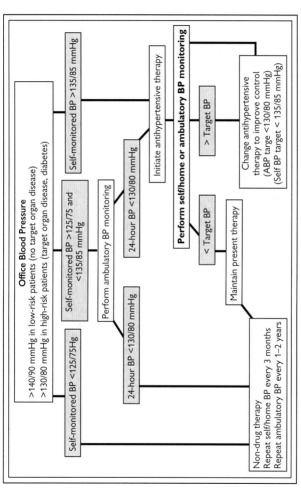

Figure 2.1 Proposed algorithm for the use of office, self-, and ambulatory BP monitoring. (Reproduced from Pickering TG, White WB; American Society of Hypertension Writing Group: ASH position paper: Home and ambulatory blood pressure monitoring. When and how to use self (home) and ambulatory blood pressure monitoring. *J Am Soc Hypertension* 2008;2:119–124, with permission from Elsevier.)

the effectiveness of complex pharmacotherapy.[27] Ambulatory BP monitoring is the only method currently available to monitor BP during sleep and to obtain accurate assessment of the morning BP surge and the circadian variability of the BP. Nocturnal BP has been strongly related to CV outcomes,[27,31] perhaps to even a greater extent than daytime, awake BP. Patterns of nocturnal BP behavior have been characterized based on the change in sleep pressure relative to the awake, daytime pressure. For example, individuals whose BP declines by more than 10% during sleep compared to the awake period are referred to as "dippers," while those lacking this 10% decline are termed "non-dippers." There are also individuals whose BP is higher at night than during the day; these have been referred to as "risers" or "reverse dippers." Individuals whose nocturnal BP is the highest have the worse clinical outcomes.[27,31,32]

Another important use of ambulatory BP measurement is in the evaluation of the surge in morning BP. The level of morning rise in BP has also been related to future CV events. The morning surge has been calculated as the difference between the 2-hour post-awakening SBP and the 2-hour pre-awakening sleep SBP. Patients who have a surge of more than 25 to 30 mm Hg have enhanced CV risk, particularly cerebrovascular events.[33]

Medical History for the Diagnosis of the Hypertensive Patient

After the diagnosis of HTN has been established by precise BP measurements as outlined above, further evaluation for all CV risk factors must be done. A comprehensive assessment of CV risk helps to guide management and determine BP goals and aids in selection of appropriate classes of antihypertensive therapy based on compelling comorbid disorders.

The medical history will provide a significant proportion of the information needed to assess CV risk. Relevant past medical history includes evaluation for comorbid risk factors, including type 1 or type 2 diabetes mellitus, dyslipidemia, obesity, smoking history, diet and exercise regimen, and the presence of vascular disease, including coronary artery disease, congestive heart failure, chronic kidney disease, stroke, and cardiac arrhythmias. In addition, it is helpful to characterize non-CV diseases that may either be associated with HTN or interfere with the treatment of the disease, such as bronchial asthma, chronic lung diseases (COPD), thyroid disorders, psychiatric diseases (anxiety and depression), and rheumatologic illnesses, particularly those that might require nonsteroidal anti-inflammatory drugs, corticosteroids, or disease-modifying agents known to raise the BP.

Characterization of the family history is relevant for the assessment of the newly diagnosed hypertensive patient. A family history of early-onset HTN or early CV disease (first-degree relative male <55 and/or female <65) is an important risk factor that will aid in clinical decision-making and possible evaluation for the underlying cause of HTN. The goal and intensity of therapy should be adjusted according to the overall CV risk assessment.

Evaluation for secondary causes of HTN is discussed in Chapter 5. Briefly, in the history of a newly diagnosed patient with HTN, the major secondary forms of HTN can be considered (Table 2.3). Proper evaluation for primary or secondary hyperaldosteronism may include a review of a history of potassium deficiency (with or without diuretic therapy), myalgias, and muscle weakness, and/or a history of antihypertensive drug resistance. Patients with renovascular disease are often more severely hypertensive, have a history of early- or late-onset HTN, and may also be resistant to antihypertensive therapies. These patients often have a history of other vascular diseases, smoking, and renal insufficiency. Patients with adrenergic excess syndromes causing HTN (pheochromocytoma and paragangliomas) are rare, but most are symptomatic with symptoms and signs of increased activity of the sympathetic nervous system.

Physical Exam

A thorough physical exam is essential in the diagnosis of a patient with HTN. The physical exam should include accurate measurement and recording of the BP, evaluation of general appearance, height, weight, waist circumference, calculation of the body mass index (BMI), fat distribution and skin changes. The physical exam must also include evaluation for evidence of target organ damage (Table 2.4). The funduscopic exam is of utmost importance in assessing for target organ damage and for risk stratification. While the funduscopic exam is of low yield in early HTN, the presence of arteriovenous nicking or arteriolar narrowing suggests a history of more prolonged or uncontrolled HTN. Flame hemorrhages, exudates, and papilledema indicate severe, accelerated, or malignant forms of HTN. Wong et al. demonstrated a progressive risk of stroke, coronary disease, and mortality as the degree of hypertensive retinopathy progressed.[34] The presence and degree of retinopathy is ideally evaluated with a dilated pupil; however, routine funduscopic examination can be performed in the physician's office without the need for dilation. The presence and degree of hypertensive retinopathy is classified from none to malignant (Table 2.5).

The CV exam is essential in the evaluation of new patients and includes determination of cardiac rate and rhythm, auscultation of the heart, and evaluation of the peripheral pulses. Determination of the point of maximal cardiac impulse (PMI) offers clues to the presence or absence of left ventricular hypertrophy (LVH). It is best performed in the left lateral decubitus position—a PMI located left of the midclavicular line and/or a sustained forceful impulse may suggest the presence of LVH. Auscultation of a loud brisk first heart sound (S1) associated with a brisk carotid upstroke also suggests the presence of a hyperdynamic and possibly enlarged left ventricle. It is common for older hypertensive patients to have an early systolic ejection murmur heard at both the apex and the base, suggesting aortic sclerosis or stenosis. There may be an associated systolic click that results from the expansion of a dilated aortic

Table 2.3 Secondary Causes of Hypertension						
Biochemical	Endocrine	Monogenetic	Vascular	Medication-Induced	Drugs of Abuse	Other
Hyperaldosteronism	Hyperthyroidism/ Hypothyroidism	Liddle syndrome	Renovascular hypertension	Corticosteroids	Nicotine	Chronic kidney disease
Pheochromocytoma/ Paraganglioma	Cushing syndrome	Gordon syndrome (pseudo-hypoaldosteronism type II)	Coarctation of the aorta	Antidepressants Monoamine oxidase inhibitors Tricyclic antidepressants Serotonin inhibitors	Alcohol	Obstructive sleep apnea
Glucocorticoid remediable aldosteronism	Congenital adrenal hyperplasia	Syndrome of apparent mineralocorticoid excess		Cyclosporine	Cocaine	
		Mineralocorticoid receptor mutations (hypertension of pregnancy)		Tacrolimus	Amphetamines	
				Over-the-counter medications Nonsteroidal anti-inflammatory drugs Decongestants (pseudoephedrine)		

Table 2.4 Physical Exam Requirements in Assessment of Hypertension

Organ System	Physical Finding
HEENT	Funduscopic exam for arterial/venous assessment, palpate thyroid, assess for venous distention, auscultation of carotid arteries
Cardiovascular	Palpate maximal impulse, auscultate for abnormal heart sounds, murmurs, cardiac rhythm, palpate vascular pulses
Respiratory	Rhonchi, rales, wheezing suggestive of bronchospasm or pulmonary vascular congestion
Abdomen	Palpate for renal masses, auscultate for aortic and renal bruits
Extremities	Peripheral pulse assessment, edema
Neurologic	Strength, symmetry, reflexes, cognitive function

Table 2.5 Classification of Hypertensive Retinopathy on the Basis of Recent Population-Based Data

Grade of Retinopathy	Retinal Signs	Systemic Associations*
None	No detectable signs	None
Mild	Generalized arteriolar narrowing, focal arteriolar narrowing, arteriovenous nicking, opacity ("copper wiring") of arteriolar wall, or a combination of these signs	Modest association with risk of clinical stroke, subclinical stroke, coronary heart disease, and death
Moderate	Hemorrhage (blot, dot, or flame-shaped), microaneurysm, cotton-wool spot, hard exudates, or a combination of these signs	Strong association with risk of clinical stroke, subclinical stroke, cognitive decline, and death from cardiovascular causes
Malignant	Signs of moderate retinopathy plus swelling of the optic disk†	Strong association with death

* A modest association is defined as an odds ratio of greater than 1 but less than 2. A strong association is defined as an odds ratio of 2 or greater.

† Anterior ischemic optic neuropathy, characterized by unilateral swelling of the optic disk, visual loss, and sectorial visual-field loss, should be ruled out.

(Reproduced with permission from Wong TY, Mitchell P. Hypertensive retinopathy. *N Engl J Med* 2004;351:2310–2317. Copyright © 2004 Massachusetts Medical Society. All rights reserved.)

root. When a systolic murmur is appreciated, evaluation for the possibility of LV outflow tract obstruction (hypertensive hypertrophic cardiomyopathy), by performing a Valsalva maneuver, is advisable. The use of direct vasodilators that induce reflex tachycardia or diuretics that reduce venous return to the heart may worsen the outflow obstruction and may need to be avoided. The early diastolic murmur of aortic regurgitation may indicate the presence of a dilated aortic root and not an anatomic abnormality; however, in such cases echocardiography would be advisable for confirmation. Finally, assessment of the carotid, femoral, and distal extremity pulses may provide clues to the presence of vascular damage or a secondary etiology of the HTN. Presence of a radial-femoral pulse delay might suggest coarctation of the aorta, especially in a younger patient. Weak or absent lower extremity pulses compared to the femoral pulses suggest a diagnosis of peripheral vascular disease, which is associated with enhanced CV risk. Auscultation and palpation of the carotid pulses may provide insight into the presence of a hyperdynamic CV system, and a carotid bruit may be due to a hemodynamically significant stenosis of the common or internal carotid artery, a risk factor for future stroke.

Conclusions

As a result of a comprehensive physical exam, identification of possible underlying or secondary causes of HTN may be made. For example, the presence of hirsutism may suggest congenital adrenal hyperplasia (11-B-hydroxylase deficiency); truncal obesity, facial plethora, and abdominal striae may raise the suspicion of Cushing syndrome. Hepatomegaly, spider angiomata, and palmar erythema could indicate alcohol abuse as an underlying cause of treatment-resistant HTN. Presence of elevated BPs in the upper extremities but not in the lower extremities may be due to coarctation of the aorta. The body habitus of a patient (obese, short neck, large tonsils, redundant uvular tissue) along with a proper medical history could indicate obstructive sleep apnea. Auscultation of an abdominal bruit might suggest renovascular HTN due to a high-grade renal artery stenosis. Hence, a comprehensive physical exam often can help in determining the laboratory or imaging evaluation requirements of the hypertensive patient.

References

1. Chobanian AV, Bakris GL, Black HR, et al.; National Heart, Lung, and Blood Institute Joint National Committee on Prevention, Detection, Evaluation, and Treatment of High Blood Pressure; National High Blood Pressure Education Program Coordinating Committee. *JAMA* 2003;21:289:2560–2572.

2. Lewington S, Clarke R, Qizilbash N, Peto R, Collins R. Age-specific relevance of usual blood pressure to vascular mortality: A meta-analysis of individual data for one million adults in 61 prospective studies. Prospective Studies Collaboration. *Lancet* 2002;360:1903–1913.

3. Cutler JA, Sorlie PD, Wolz M, Thom T, Fields LE, Roccella EJ. Trends in hypertension prevalence, awareness, treatment, and control rates in United States adults between 1988–1994 and 1999–2004. *Hypertension* 2008;52:818–827.

4. Egan BM, Zhao Y, Axon RN. US trends in prevalence, awareness, treatment, and control of hypertension, 1988–2008 *JAMA* 2010;303:2043–2050.

5. Gu Q, Dillon CF, Burt VL, Gillum RF. Association of hypertension treatment and control with all-cause and cardiovascular disease mortality among US adults with hypertension. *Am J Hypertens* 2010;23:38–45.

6. Thavarajah S, White WB, Mansoor GA. Terminal digit bias in a specialty HTN faculty practice. *J Hum Hypertens* 2003;17:819–822.

7. Nietert PJ, Wessel AM, Feifer C, Ornstein SM. Effect of terminal digit preference on blood pressure measurement and treatment in primary care. *Am J Hypertens* 2006;19:147–152.

8. Manning DM, Kuchirka C, Kaminski J. Miscuffing: inappropriate blood pressure cuff application. *Circulation* 1983;8:101–106.

9. Harrison WN, Lancashire RJ, Marshall TP. Variation in recorded blood pressure terminal digit bias in general practice. *J Hum Hypertens* 2008;22:163–167.

10. Wingfield D, Cooke J, Thijs LJ, et al., on behalf of the Syst-Eur Investigators. Terminal digit preference and single number preference in the Syst-Eur trial: influence of quality control. *Blood Press Monit* 2002;7:169–177.

11. Cavallini MC, Roman MJ, Blank SG et al. Association of the auscultatory gap with vascular disease in hypertensive patients. *Ann Intern Med* 1996;124:877–883.

12. Myers MG. Automated blood pressure measurement for diagnosing hypertension. *Blood Press Monit* 2007;12:405–406.

13. Myers MG, Godwin M. Automated measurements of blood pressure in routine clinical practice. *J Clin Hypertens* 2007;9:267–270.

14. Myers MG, Valdivieso M, Kiss A. Use of automated office blood pressure measurement to reduce the white coat response. *J Hypertens* 2009;27:280–286.

15. White WB. Ambulatory blood-pressure monitoring in clinical practice. *N Engl J Med* 2003;348:2377–2378.

16. Gustavsen PH, Hoegholm A, Bank LE, Kristensen KS. White coat hypertension is a cardiovascular risk factor: a 10-year follow-up study. *J Hum Hypertens* 2003;17:811–817.

17. Yarrows SA, Staessen JA. How to use ambulatory blood pressure monitors in clinical practice. *Am J Hypertens* 2002;15:93–96.

18. Pickering TG, Hall JE, Appel LJ, et al. Recommendations for blood pressure measurement in humans and experimental animals: Part 1: Blood pressure measurement in humans: a statement for professionals from the Subcommittee of Professional and Public Education of the American Heart Association Council on High Blood Pressure Research. *Circulation* 2005;111:697–716.

19. Mule G, Caimi G, Cottone S, et al. Value of home blood pressures as predictor of target organ damage in mild arterial hypertension. *J Cardiovasc Risk* 2002;9123–129.

20. Pickering TG, Miller NH, Ogedegbe G, et al.; American Heart Association; American Society of HTN; Preventive Cardiovascular Nurses Association. Call to action on use and reimbursement for home blood pressure monitoring: a joint statement by the American Heart Association, American Society of Hypertension, and the Preventive Cardiovascular Nurses' Association. *Hypertension* 2008;52:1–9.

21. O'Brien E, Petrie J, Littler WA et al. The British HTN Society protocol for the evaluation of blood pressure measuring devices. *J Hypertens* 1993;11:S43–S63.

22. Association for the Advancement of Medical Instrumentation. *American National Standard: electronic or automated sphygmomanometers*. ANSI/AAMI SP 10–1992. Arlington, VA: Association for the Advancement of Medical Instrumentation, 1993:40.

23. Bombelli M, Sega R, Facchetti R, et al. Prevalence and clinical significance of a greater ambulatory versus office blood pressure ("reversed white coat" condition) in a general population. *J Hypertens* 2005;23:513–520.

24. Bobrie G, Genes N, Vaur L, et al. Is "isolated home" HTN as opposed to "isolated office" HTN a sign of greater cardiovascular risk? *Arch Intern Med* 2001;161:2205–2211.

25. Sterigou GS, Skeva II, Baibas NM, et al. Diagnosis of HTN using home or ambulatory blood pressure monitoring: comparison with conventional strategy based on repeated clinic blood pressure measurements. *J Hypertens* 2000;18:1745–1751.

26. Stergiou GS, Zourbaki AS, Skeva II, Mountokalakis TD. White coat effect detected using self-monitoring of blood pressure at home: comparison with ambulatory blood pressure. *Am J Hypertens* 1998;11:820–827.

27. Pickering TG, White WB; American Society of HTN Writing Group: ASH position paper: Home and ambulatory blood pressure monitoring. When and how to use self (home) and ambulatory blood pressure monitoring. *J Am Soc Hypertens* 2008;2:119–124.

28. Sega R, Facchetti R, Bombelli M, et al. Prognostic value of ambulatory and home blood pressures compared with office blood pressure in the general population: follow-up results from the Pressioni Arteriose Monitorate e Loro Associazioni (PAMELA) study. *Circulation* 2005;111:1777–1783.

29. Clement DL, De Buyzere ML, De Bacquer DA, et al., for the Office versus Ambulatory Pressure Study Investigators. Prognostic value of ambulatory blood-pressure recordings in patients with treated HTN. *N Engl J Med* 2003;348:2407–2415.

30. Ohkubo T, Asayama K, Kikuya M, et al. Prediction of ischemic and hemorrhagic stroke by self-measured blood pressure at home: the Ohasama study. *Blood Press Monit* 2004;9:315–320.

31. Sierra A, Redon J, Banegas J, et al.; Spanish Society of HTN Ambulatory Blood Pressure Monitoring Registry Investigators: Prevalence and factors associated with circadian blood pressure patterns in hypertensive patients. *Hypertension* 2009;53:466–472.

32. Pickering TG, Shimbo D, Haas D. Ambulatory blood-pressure monitoring. *N Engl J Med* 2006;354:2368–2374.

33. Li Y, Thijs L, Hansen TW, et al., for the International Database on Ambulatory Blood Pressure Monitoring in Relation to Cardiovascular Outcomes Investigators. Prognostic value of the morning blood pressure surge in 5645 subjects from 8 populations. *Hypertension* 2010;55:1040–1048.

34. Wong TY, Mitchell P. Hypertensive retinopathy. *N Engl J Med* 2004;351: 2310–2317.

Chapter 3

Laboratory and Diagnostic Procedures

Clarence E. Grim, MS, MD

The laboratory evaluation in the new hypertensive patient has five objectives (modified from JNC 1 thru 7 and likely 8):[1]

1. To assess the two major dietary factors that are driving the patient's BP to unhealthy levels: excess intake of sodium (Na) and deficient intake of potassium (K)
2. To screen for known curable causes of high BP
3. To detect the three CV risk factors that affect prognosis and will guide choice and goals of treatment:
   a. Hyperlipidemia
   b. Diabetes mellitus
   c. Impaired renal function/renal disease

4. To detect other disease processes that may affect clinician recommendations for lifestyle changes (alcohol) and/or choice of drugs
5. To begin/supplement the patient's personal home health record. Patients must be partners in the management of their high BP for the rest of their life. It is not likely you will be their physician for this entire time, so a record of your testing will prevent them from having to have redundant tests in the future.

Although the detailed testing strategy will depend on the patient's history and the results of the physical examination, a set of basic tests should be performed in all patients at their first visit. It should be noted that target normal values for the recommend laboratory tests are not being given here, as each testing laboratory has its own normal values, and clinicians should always use these rather than published normal values.

Introduction

The goal of laboratory testing (urine and blood) is to help the clinician and patient answer the following questions:

1. Is high Na and low K intake the likely cause of the patient's HTN?
2. Does the patient have a genetic or secondary cause of HTN for which there is a specific therapy or cure?

3. What other CVD risk factors need to be addressed in the treatment plan (hyperlipidemia, diabetes, renal disease)?
   a. What should be the treatment goal for the BP?
   b. Does the patient have a compelling indication for a specific drug regimen (hyperlipidemia, diabetes, renal disease)?
4. Are there other major illnesses that may be affecting the patient's BP as well as our treatment plan?

By giving patients a copy of test results, clinicians can help them begin their home health care record system, which will play an important role in helping them live a healthier and longer life over the next 10, 20, 30, or 40 years.

Background

In interpreting the results of basic lab tests, the clinician must consider the most common physiologic forces that are driving the patient's BP to unhealthy levels. If the cause can be discerned, then the treatment can be targeted to that cause. This will save both the clinician and the patient months or years of frustration in trying to manage the most common chronic disease seen: elevated BP.

Testing for Causes

Although most patients (60%) will NOT have a currently known cause for their HTN, recent research has explored the known causes of HTN for which there are specific methods of treatment or cure. Thus, a great number of patients today will have a specific treatable cause that will simplify the task of getting their BP to goal with as few medications and side effects as possible.

The three major advances in the clinical laboratory testing for causes of high BP today are diet assessment (estimate diet Na and K intake), physiologic measures of BP control systems (the aldosterone-renin-angiotensin and catecholamine system), and genetic testing.

Diet

The key environmental force driving a patient's BP to unhealthy levels is consuming too much NaCl and not enough K, which forces the patient's inherited pressure natriuresis system to increase the BP to maintain body sodium homeostasis.[2,3]

Renin-Angiotensin-Aldosterone System

A major advance in clinical laboratory testing is the universal ability to measure renin and aldosterone to screen for the most common non-dietary causes of HTN: the various forms of primary aldosteronism (high aldosterone/low renin)[4] and renal artery stenosis (not low renin) and pheochromocytoma (catecholamines).

Genes

The major genetic (familial) causes of high BP also involve the manner in which the kidney retains sodium (and excretes K). Recent advances have made it possible to test for these specific causes (see chapter on genetic causes of HTN). These genetic tests are not yet available through most laboratories but may be in the near future.

Test Selection

The patient history and physical exam must guide your laboratory testing. Focused testing will enable the clinician to answer the following questions.

Is the Patient's Dietary Na/K Intake Playing a Role in the HTN?

The answer is almost certainly yes. In addition, many patients are asking, "Doctor, is there anything I can do to avoid drugs to control my blood pressure?" Your answer should be, "Yes! If you can change your eating pattern to that of the DASH eating plan (Dietary Approaches to Stop Hypertension),[3] you may well be able to avoid any BP meds" (especially if the patient is at stage 1 HTN [about 40% of all patients with HTN]). Patients at stage 2 HTN may find they need fewer drugs if they can follow the DASH plan successfully.

The most effective way to lower BP without drugs is to recommend a DASH eating program. This is also the easiest lifestyle change to monitor; all it takes is an estimate of the Na and K in the patient's urine. Therefore, at the first visit I recommend a simple spot urine test for Na, K, and creatinine (albumin levels should also be measured in this same urine sample). If the urine contains more Na than K (mM/L), then the patient is not consuming the recommended Na/K ratio of the DASH eating plan (see Chapter 4 on DASH). The spot urine analysis can be used to give patients feedback on their Na intake by using the equation developed by Mann et al.[5] If excessive Na is being consumed (>1,500 mg/day) and/or not enough K is being consumed (>4,700 mg/day). it is very likely that a major contributor to your patient's HTN is excess Na and suboptimal K intake. Armed with this information you can now recommend to patients that by following the DASH diet for the next 2 weeks (rigidly using Chapter 9 in the DASH book[3] and measuring their home BP (see Chapter 2 on home measurement), they will be able to quickly determine the role of diet in their unhealthy BP. As most of the BP effect of the low-Na DASH diet is apparent by 2 weeks, you and your patient can quickly test this before beginning any medical therapy.

Based on research by Dr. S.J. Mann's group at Cornell, one of the best ways to document patients' salt intake is to measure Na and creatinine in a spot urine analysis. After adjusting for their age, gender, and weight, you can give them feedback that they are or are not at the DASH goal. The final conversion formula is not yet published.[6]

A spot urine K analysis can also be performed. By looking at the Na/K ratio (in mM/L) you can inform patients that they are or are not "DASHing." The

DASH guidelines are not being followed if there is not more K than Na in the urine (in mM/L). This can be also be used at follow-up visits to monitor compliance with your recommendations for Na and K intake.

Does the Patient Have a Genetic or Other Primary Cause of HTN?

If your patient's family history is strong, then you must suspect one of the known familial causes of HTN (see Chapters).

What Other CVD Risk Factors Need to Be Addressed in the Treatment Plan, and How Will They Affect the Choice of Drugs and Goal BP?

Because of the many causes of HTN and the wide variety of nutritional and pharmacologic agents that may need to be used for BP control, the basic testing panel not only screens for possible reversible or specific treatable causes of HTN, it also assesses the need for specific BP goals (<130/80 mm Hg in diabetes mellitus or renal disease), quantifies the damage that HTN has done to the kidneys (urinary protein/creatinine ratio), and classifies other CVD risk factors that will need to be addressed to maximize the patient's short- and long-term health. These are summarized in Table 3.1.

The only reliable way to assess Na and K intake is to perform a timed urinalysis measuring Na, K, and creatinine levels. This same timed urinalysis will give you the most accurate estimate of renal function (glomerular filtration rate). The closer to a 24-hour urine collection, the better. Because of the difficulty in collecting a 24-hour urine, however, it is preferred to do an overnight urine for this assessment, as it is easier to collect. Have the patient urinate when he or she goes to bed and discard this urine. Record this time. Set the collection bottle on the closed toilet seat. This is a good reminder that urine is being collected in case the patient gets up to urinate at night. Collect all urine during the night and the first voided urine on arising. Record this time. Now you have a timed urine collection. This can be converted (more or less) to a 24-hour estimate of Na and K intake and creatinine clearance. If you suspect pheochromocytoma or Cushing syndrome, the sleep urine is also the best urine test to measure catecholamines or urinary free cortisol, as sleep produces the lowest excretion of both.

The second task is to do (and review) the basic battery of recommended tests (ever since JNC 1) to screen for causes of HTN and to assess the patient's overall CV risk so you can decide if the patient needs to be treated with something other than a diuretic as the first effort to lower the BP if the DASH program does not get his or her BP to goal.

1. Renal causes: A clean-catch midstream urine for dipstick screening and microscopic examination, microalbuminuria, BUN/creatinine, and estimated glomerular filtration rate.
2. Testing for diabetes: Recent revisions of the testing for diabetes recommends that a HbA1c be obtained on a fasting sample, along with plasma glucose.[7]
3. Complete blood count (hematocrit): Polycythemia or anemia may affect BP. Caution if low white count with certain BP drugs.

Table 3.1 Clinical Laboratory Testing in Hypertension

1. Is the patient eating excess Na and/or deficient K? Spot urine Na, K, creatinine.
2. Does the patient have a secondary cause of HTN?
    a. Renal? Urinalysis, BUN/creatinine, urine albuminuria/creatinine ratio
    b. Adrenal?
        i. Low K and/or diabetes: Suspect one of the forms of primary aldosterone excess. Aldosterone/renin ratio.
        ii. "Spells" of HTH, headaches, tachycardia: Suspect pheochromocytoma. Urine catecholamines.
    c. Genetic HTN: Plasma K is often a clue to this group. Aldosterone/renin ratio.
        i. Low K?
1. Inherited ENaC HTN (Liddle syndrome)
2. Inherited renal 17B hydroxylase deficiency (apparent mineralocorticoid excess)
3. Pregnancy HTN due to activation mutation for ENaC
        ii. High K? Inherited hypertension hyperkalemia syndromes
    d. Hypercalcemia: Hyperparathyroidism?
    e. Uric Acid: gout in the future?
    f. CBC: microangiopathic hemolytic anemia syndrome, polycythemia, anemia
3. Does the patient have other CVD risk factors that must be addressed?
    a. Diabetes? HbA1c, glucose, albumin/creatinine
    b. Hyperlipidemia? Lipid panel/TSH
    c. Renal disease? Albumin/creatinine
4. Do the laboratory results tell me I need a lower BP treatment goal? <130/80 in office or <125/75 home.
    a. Diabetes
    b. Renal disease
5. Does the patient have laboratory evidence of target organ damage?
    a. Renal: Glomerular filtration rate/proteinuria
6. Does the patient have other problems that I must consider in recommending lifestyle changes (alcohol intake)? Liver disease.
7. Does the patient have reasons I should use specific antihypertensives? Congestive heart failure, diabetes, renal disease.

4. Plasma electrolytes: A common problem is that many laboratories do not follow guidelines that ensure an accurate K level (no fist clenching; draw electrolytes last and ideally after release of the tourniquet). Insist that the lab you send your patient to follow these guidelines, and tell your patient how you want the blood drawn. A low K in the absence of diuretic therapy is strongly suggestive of the many known causes of HTN that lower K, including many inherited causes of HTN. A low sodium suggests secondary aldosteronism, especially renovascular HTN, or a side effect of diuretics, especially in the elderly.

5. Creatinine clearance: Many causes of HTN are secondary to renal disease and the decreased ability to excrete salt.

6. Urinary microalbuminuria:[8] By measuring the albumin/creatinine ration in an overnight or first morning urine in your office, you can get the

best indicator of renal glomerular damage from HTN, diabetes mellitus, or atherosclerosis. The results will guide which drugs you choose to
use and will serve as a baseline for monitoring successful therapy, which
should not only lower BP but also reduce microalbuminuria.

7. Comprehensive metabolic panel: glucose, calcium, albumin/total protein,
   sodium, potassium, CO_2, chloride, BUN, creatinine, alkaline phosphatase
   (ALP), alanine amino transferase (ALT or SGPT), aspartate amino transferase (AST or SGOT), and bilirubin.

8. Lipid profile, after a 9- to 12-hour fast (always have your patient come to
   the clinic in a fasting state), that includes high-density lipoprotein cholesterol, low-density lipoprotein cholesterol, triglycerides, and if hyperlipi-
   demic TSH.

**The New Patient Has Been Controlled on Two or More BP Meds.
What Should I Test For?**

If the drugs being used are combinations of beta-blockers, ACE inhibitors,
angiotensin II receptor blockers (ARBs), or renin inhibitors, then it is likely the
patient has a low renin problem, as these drugs work poorly in this setting.[4]
Now is the time to measure plasma renin activity and plasma aldosterone and
do a 24-hour urine for Na, K, and creatinine and aldosterone.

When Should I Measure Renin and Aldosterone?

If the patient has ever had a low K or requires more than two drugs to get the
BP to goal, then it is important to rule out the most common cause of drug-
resistant HTN: primary aldosteronism in its many forms.[3] The patient does
not need to have a low K for you to suspect primary aldosteronism. Failure to
control the BP with a beta-blocker, ACE inhibitor/ARB, or low K on a diuretic
are all good clues to the presence of primary aldosteronism, as these drugs do
not work in the presence of primary adrenal aldosterone excess. Some recommend that extensive testing for identifiable causes is not indicated unless BP
control is not achieved. However, because many drugs that are used to try to
get BP under control will fail in patients with various causes of HTN, and may
even make the HTN worse,[9] I recommend measuring renin and aldosterone
(see Chapter XX for interpretation) before starting therapy in all stage 2 HTN
or drug-resistant patients.

Summary

Table 3.2 summarizes recommended clinical laboratory testing needed to diagnose, classify, and manage the patient with high BP. By basing "routine" laboratory testing in the new hypertensive patient on a detailed history and physical
examination, you will be able to take advantage of the power of clinical laboratory testing in your individual patient management. By answering key questions
about the patient's laboratory results, you will be able to design a comprehensive short- and long-term treatment plan and answer the following questions:

Table 3.2 Recommended Clinical Laboratory Testing Needed to Diagnose, Classify, and Manage the Patient with High Blood Pressure

Source	Test	Baseline	CVD Risk?	Guide Goal BP and Rx?	Follow-up: Better or Worse with Rx or Due to Rx?
Blood	CBC	Assess causes	Yes	No	Anemias associated with several HTN drugs
	Hematocrit	Assess for polycythemia/anemia.	Yes	Yes	Yes
	WBC		Yes	No	Yes: side effects of HTN drugs
	Differential	High eosinophils	No	No	Drug allergies
	Glucose, HbA1c	Diagnose diabetes mellitus and assess CVD risk	Yes	Yes	Change with Rx for HTN
	Fasting lipid profile with TSH	Assess CVD risk. Additional Rx required.	Yes	Yes	Change with Rx for HTN. Thyroid dysfunction causing HTN.
	Liver function tests from CMP	Assess for liver disease, excess alcohol intake.	No	Yes	Drug side effects
	Calcium[1]	Hyperparathyroidism	?	?	Yes
	Uric acid[2]	Probability of developing gout	??	Yes	Yes
	TSH	Hyper- or hypothyroidism		Yes	No
	Aldosterone/renin ratio	Best way to detect causes of diseases associated with drug-resistant HTN	No	Yes	Always assess if more than 2 classes of drugs are needed or it hypokalemic ever.

(continued)

Table 3.2 (Continued)

Source	Test	Baseline	CVD Risk?	Guide Goal BP and Rx?	Follow-up: Better or Worse with Rx or Due to Rx?
Urine	Urinalysis dipstick	Protein, blood, infection	Yes	Yes	Yes
	Microscopic	Causes of renal disease	No	Yes	Yes
	Spot/sleep urine for albumin/creatinine ratio	Assess glomerular/tubular damage.	Yes	Yes	Yes
	Spot: Na, K, creatinine	Assess diet intake. Is HTN likely related to diet?	Yes:	Yes	Feedback on adherence to DASH
	Sleep or 24-hr urine Cortisol	Screen for Cushing syndrome.	No	Yes	Refer for endocrine evaluation.
	Sleep or 24-hr urine for catecholamines	Screen for pheochromocytoma if history is compatible (see Chapter 3).	No	Yes	Refer to HTN specialist.
	24-hour urine: creatinine, Na, K	Precise estimate of GFR, Na, and K intake	Yes	Yes	Yes
	24-hr urine for Na, K, aldosterone	In conjunction with aldo/renin ratio. Assess all drug-resistant HTN cases for likely primary aldosteronism.	No	Yes	Refer to HTN specialist.

[1] See Chapter 3 on secondary causes.
[2] See Chapter 3 on gout.

What lifestyle changes should I recommend? Does the patient have a secondary cause of HTN? What BP goal should I select? Which drugs should I start with? What other risk factors do I need to include in the long-term treatment plan? Providing patients with the results of this testing for their records will set the stage for their lifelong treatment plan and home medical record system.

References

1. Chobanian AV, Bakris GL, Black HR, Cushman WC, Green LA, Izzo JL Jr, Jones DW, Materson BJ, Oparil S, Wright JT Jr, Roccella EJ. The Seventh Report of the Joint National Committee on Prevention, Detection, Evaluation, and Treatment of High Blood Pressure: the JNC 7 report. *JAMA* 2003;289:2560–2572.

2. Guyton AC, Coleman TG. Quantitative analysis of the pathophysiology of hypertension. *J Am Soc Nephrol* 1999;10(10):2248–2258.

3. Moore TA, Jenkins M, Svetkey L, Pap-Hwa L, Karanja N. *DASH Diet for Hypertension*. New York: Pocket Books, Simon & Schuster, 2001.

4. Grim CE. Evolution of diagnostic criteria for primary aldosteronism: why is it more common in "drug-resistant" hypertension today? *Curr Hypertens Rep* 2004;6:485–492.

5. Mann SJ, Gerber LM. Estimation of 24-hour sodium excretion from spot urine samples. *J Clin Hypertens* 2010;12:174–180.

6. Mann SJ. Cornell University. personal communication: Jan. 21, 2011.

7. American Diabetes Association. Diagnosis and classification of diabetes mellitus. *Diabetes Care* 2010;34(Supplement 1):S62–S69.

8. Bakris GL. Microalbuminuria: what is it? Why is it important? What should be done about it? *J Clin Hypertens* 2001;3(2):99–102.

9. Alderman MH, Cohen HW, Sealey JE, Laragh JH. Pressor responses to antihypertensive drug types. *Am J Hypertens* 2010;23(9):1031–1037.

Chapter 4

Treatment of Essential Hypertension

Michael R. Lattanzio, DO and Matthew R. Weir, MD

Overview

What defines meaningful treatment of HTN? In simplistic terms, BP treatment should alter the upward slope of change of BP over time. To achieve this treatment goal, physicians must consider many variables that influence BP, principally age, ethnicity, genetics, and environmental factors. Numerous epidemiologic studies demonstrate a continuous direct relationship between adverse CV events and BP (Fig. 4.1). This provides the impetus for BP reduction strategies. Despite evidence that reducing BP reduces CV events over time, we lack objective data in terms of the optimal BP goals in different population groups, depending on age and medical comorbidity. We assume that lower BP will translate into a more substantial reduction in incident CV events, but there is a paucity of data with targeted treatment to below SBPs of 130 mm Hg, let alone below 140 mm Hg.

The treatment of HTN is challenging secondary to its largely asymptomatic and progressive nature. Moreover, the institution of therapy may engender undesirable side effects that will limit adherence and have an adverse impact on the long-term, salubrious effects of BP control. As a result of these confounding factors, BP treatment strategies must be personalized, dynamic, tolerable, and able to be implemented. We provide an evidence-based strategy for BP control in the treatment of otherwise uncomplicated essential HTN.

Non-pharmacologic Strategies

Lifestyle modifications, such as weight reduction, dietary alterations, and exercise, have consistently been shown to effectively reduce BP in short-term studies (Table 4.1). For example, in the Dietary Approaches to Stop Hypertension (DASH) study, 8 weeks of a diet of fruits, vegetables, low-fat dairy products, whole grains, poultry, fish, and nuts, with limited fats, red meat, and sweets, reduced SBP by 5.5 mm Hg.[1] A reduction in sodium intake should also be endorsed for its ability to reduce BP per se. In the DASH study, the addition of low sodium intake (<100 mmol/day) to the DASH dietary changes resulted in an additional drop in SBP of 3 mm Hg and DBP of 1.6 mm Hg.[2] Besides the

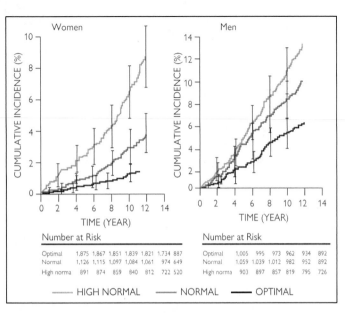

Figure 4.1 Cumulative incidence of cardiovascular events in women (Panel A) and men (Panel B) in optimal, normal, and high-normal BP categories. Optimal BP is SBP <120 mm Hg and DBP <80 mm Hg. Normal BP is SBP 120 to 129 mm Hg and DBP 80 to 84 mm Hg. High-normal BP is SBP 130 to 139 mm Hg or DBP 85 to 89 mm Hg. Vertical bars indicate 95% confidence intervals. (From Vasan RS, Larson MG, Leip EP, Evans JC, O'Donnell CJ, Kannel WB, Levy D. Impact of high-normal blood pressure on the risk of cardiovascular disease. *N Engl J Med* 2001;345:1291–1297. Copyright © 2001 Massachusetts Medical Society. All rights reserved.)

Table 4.1 Lifestyle modifications to prevent and manage hypertension

Modification	Recommendation	Anticipated Systolic Blood Pressure Reduction (mm Hg)*
Weight loss	Maintain normal body weight (body mass index 18.5–24.9 kg/m²)	5–20 mm Hg/10 kg
DASH diet	Diet rich in fruits, vegetables, low-fat dairy	8–14 mm Hg
Sodium restriction	Less than 100 mmol or 2.4 grams of sodium per day	2–8 mm Hg
Physical activity	Regular, aerobic exercise	4–9 mm Hg
Reduce alcohol consumption	Limit to 2 drinks/day in men and 1 drink/day in women	2–4 mm Hg

* = the effects of these modification of dose and time dependent, and could br greater for some individuals.

direct effect of sodium reduction on BP, sodium reduction can indirectly lower BP by enhancing the effects of most antihypertensive agents. More importantly, observational follow-up of the Trials of Hypertension Prevention (TOHP) showed that sodium reduction resulted in a 25% risk reduction for CV events over a 10- to 15-year follow-up period (Fig. 4.2).[3]

The BP reduction associated with dietary modifications can be augmented by the institution of a regular aerobic exercise routine. In epidemiologic studies, exercise was a significant independent predictor of reduced CVD events among hypertensive subjects, after adjusting for other CVD risk factors.[4] Smoking cessation should be encouraged in any hypertensive patient because it can markedly increase the risk of secondary CV complications.

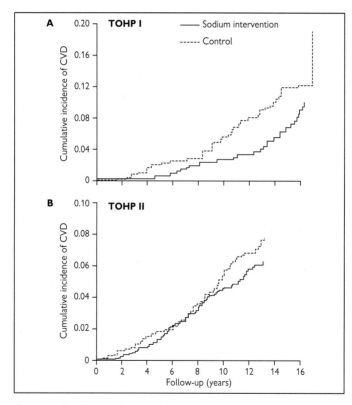

Figure 4.2 Cumulative incidence of cardiovascular disease by sodium intervention group. Panel A includes data from TOHP I and Panel B includes data from TOHP II. Net sodium restrictions in the intervention groups were 44 mmol/day and 33 mmol/day, respectively. Adjustments made for age, sex, and clinic. (Reproduced from Cook NR, Cutler JA, Obarzanek E, Buring JE, Rexrode KM, Kumanyika SK, Appel LJ, Whelton PK. Long-term effects of dietary sodium reduction on cardiovascular disease outcomes: observational follow-up of the trials of hypertension prevention (TOHP). *BMJ* 2007;334:885–888, with permission from BMJ Publishing Group Ltd.)

To date, there are few randomized controlled data that non-pharmacologic modalities can reduce CV events in the essential HTN population. In general, diminished compliance with non-pharmacologic therapies over time may limit their utility as a long-term strategy for BP control.

Pharmacologic Strategies

Strategy Overview

Pharmacologic agents that are suitable for the initial management of uncomplicated essential HTN include thiazide diuretics, long-acting calcium-channel blockers, and angiotensin-converting enzyme (ACE) inhibitors/angiotensin receptor blockers (ARBs). These specific medications have demonstrated an ability to reduce CV events within the general population. A global assessment of all factors contributing to an individual's BP control should be performed to improve the likelihood of long-term success. Short of a compelling indication, drug tolerability and efficacy should dictate the antihypertensive agent chosen for initial therapy. An algorithm for BP control in the uncomplicated essential hypertensive patient is shown in Figure 4.3.

Renin-Angiotensin-Aldosterone System (RAAS) Blockade

There are convincing data for the use of ACE inhibitors/ARBs for essential HTN in individuals with a compelling indication, specifically diabetes, proteinuric kidney disease, and heart failure. The role of ACE inhibitors/ARBs as a preferred treatment for uncomplicated essential HTN is less well defined. As will be discussed, one of the advantages of these therapies is that they are well tolerated and their use is not associated with a dose-related increase in side effects.

BP management with ACE inhibitors should be strongly considered in patients at high risk for CV disease (age >55 years who have evidence of vascular disease plus one other CV risk factor). The Heart Outcomes Prevention (HOPE) trial assessed the role of an ACE inhibitor, ramipril, in patients who were at high risk for CV events but who did not have overt left ventricular dysfunction or heart failure.[5] Almost 50% of the patients included in the HOPE trial were hypertensive at entry. In this study, ramipril significantly reduced the rates of death, myocardial infarction (MI), and stroke in a broad range of high-risk patients who were not known to have a low ejection fraction or heart failure.[5] The HOPE trial provides strong support for the institution of ACE inhibitor therapy among individuals at high risk for CV events.

Can the treatment of essential HTN with ARBs reduce the incidence of future CV events? In the Losartan Intervention for Endpoint Reduction (LIFE) trial, ARB therapy with losartan was more effective than beta-blockade with atenolol in reducing CV morbidity and death in patients with essential HTN and evidence of LVH.[6] In the Study on Cognition and Prognosis in the Elderly (SCOPE), ARB therapy was associated with a significant reduction in nonfatal stroke compared to diuretic therapy in mildly hypertensive elderly patients.[7]

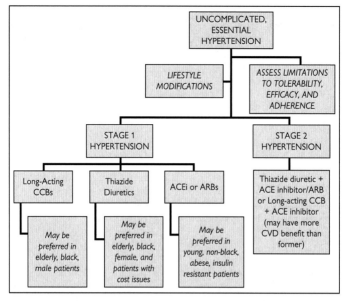

Figure 4.3 Treatment algorithm for the management of uncomplicated essential HTN. The management of uncomplicated essential HTN requires a global assessment of the patient to identify limitations to tolerability, efficacy, and adherence. Lifestyle modifications should be instituted for all patients with essential HTN. Stage I HTN (SBP 140 to 159 mm Hg or DBP 90 to 99 mm Hg) requires initiation of therapy with monotherapy (long-acting CCB, thiazide diuretic, or ACE inhibitor/ARB). Stage II HTN (SBP >160 mm Hg or DBP >100 mm Hg) requires multiple agents. The appropriate monotherapy and dual therapy depends on many factors, including age, sex, race, and financial situation.

Interestingly, these ARB trials demonstrated a significant relative risk reduction in the incidence of diabetes among the general population that may translate into a reduction of future CV events.

A substantial number of CV and kidney disease outcome trials provide evidence that using either ACE inhibitors or ARBs, in conjunction with improved BP control, provides an incremental ~20% relative risk reduction benefit compared to other antihypertensive therapies. One larger clinical trial, the Ongoing Telmisartan Alone and in Combination with Ramipril Global Endpoints Trial (ONTARGET), demonstrated therapeutic equivalence between the ACE inhibitor and the ARB on the reduction of all vascular events.[8] These studies are largely conducted in patients with more vascular disease and CV risk factors, and thus are indicative of a secondary prevention benefit. What is not known is whether these drugs will provide a primary prevention benefit, compared to other therapies, started early in the course of hypertensive treatment.

Another newer strategy for lowering BP is the direct renin inhibitor (DRI). This therapy is biochemically distinct from the ACE inhibitor/ARB because it

Table 4.2 Antihypertensive Agents

Class	Subclass	Drug	Usual Dose Range (mg/day)	Usual Dosing Frequency
ACE Inhibitors		Benazepril	10–40	1–2
		Captopril	25–100	2–3
		Enalapril	5–40	1–2
		Fosinopril	10–40	1
		Lisinopril	10–40	1
		Moexipril	7.5–30	1–2
		Perindopril	4–8	1
		Quinapril	10–80	1–2
		Ramipril	2.5–20	1–2
		Trandolapril	1–4	1
Alpha 1 Blockers		Doxazosin	1–16	1
		Prazosin	2–20	2–3
		Terazosin	1–20	1–2
ARBs		Azilsartan	40–80	1
		Candesartan	8–32	1–2
		Eprosartan	400–800	1–2
		Irbesartan	150–300	1
		Losartan	25–100	1–2
		Olmesartan	20–40	1
		Telmisartan	20–80	1
		Valsartan	80–320	1
Beta Blockers	Cardioselective	Atenolol	25–100	1
		Betaxolol	5–20	1
		Bisoprolol	2.5–10	1
		Metoprolol	100–400	2
	Nonselective	Nadolol	40–120	1
		Propranolol	160–480	2
		Timolol	10–40	1
	Intrinsic Sympathomimetic Activity	Acebutolol	200–800	2
		Carteolol	2.5–10	1
		Penbutolol	10–40	1
		Pindolol	10–60	3
	Mixed apha/beta blockers	Carvedilol	12.5–50	2
		Labetolol	200–800	2
	Cardioselective and vasodilatory	Nebivolol	5–20	1
Calcium Channel Blockers	Dihydropyridines	Amlodipine	2.5–10	1
		Felodipine	2.5–20	1
		Isradipine	2.5–10	2

Table 4.2 (Continued)				
Class	**Subclass**	**Drug**	**Usual Dose Range (mg/day)**	**Usual Dosing Frequency**
		Nicardipine	60–120	2
		Nifedipine	30–60	1
		Nisoldipine	10–40	1
	Non-dihydropyridines	Diltiazem	180–240	2
		Verapamil	80–320	1–2
Central alpha 2 Inhibitors		Clonidine	0.1–0.8	2
		Methyldopa	250–1000	2
Direct Arterial Vasodilators		Minoxidil	2.5–80	2–3
		Hydralazine	25–100	2–4
Direct Renin Inhibitors		Aliskiren	150–300	1
Diuretics	Thiazides	Chlorthalidone	6.25–25	1
		Hydrochlorothiazide	12.5–25	1
		Indapamide	1.25–2.5	1
		Metolazone	0.5–1	1
	Loop	Bumetanide	0.5–4	2
		Furosemide	20–80	2
		Torsemide	5–10	1
	Potassium sparing	Amiloride	5–10	1–2
		Triamterene	50–100	1–2
	Aldosterone Antagonists	Eplerenone	50–100	1–2
		Spironolactone	25–50	1–2
Peripheral Adrenergic Antagonist		Reserpine	0.1–0.25	1

blocks the first step in the RAAS cascade, and neutralizes plasma renin activity. Aliskiren is a DRI that effectively lowers BP in hypertensive individuals. Aliskiren has demonstrated potential benefit in diabetic nephropathy patients given its ability to further reduce proteinuria when combined with other RAAS blocking agents.[9] There are no completed studies yet demonstrating the cardiovascular benefit of aliskiren either alone or as part of combination therapy in individuals with essential HTN; however, these studies are underway. The expense of DRIs may limit their generalized use, compared to generic ACE inhibitors.

Although they are generally well tolerated, cough was the most common reason for the discontinuation of ACE inhibitors in randomized controlled trials. Cough is not a frequent side effect associated with therapy with ARBs or

DRIs; therefore, they are suitable substitutes for ACE inhibitors in the cough-intolerant patient. Angioedema is a rare, life-threatening, adverse drug event that requires immediate cessation of ACE inhibitors. From a cost perspective, ACE inhibitors have the advantage over ARBs given the availability of generic formulations. As generic versions of RAAS blockers become available, there may be less financial incentive to choose diuretics over ACE inhibitors/ARBs as initial monotherapy.

The response to RAAS blockade may not be stereotypical across different populations. For example, studies have consistently shown that RAAS block-ade may be more efficacious in achieving BP control in the higher-renin, less volume-dependent, hypertensive states that are typical of younger and non-black patients. Higher doses of RAAS blockers are often required to lower BP in patients with a lower renin phenotype. Physicians should be cognizant of the differential response to RAAS blockers so appropriate doses can be employed to avoid delaying the achievement of meaningful BP reduction.

Diuretic Therapy

Diuretic therapy reduces BP when administered as monotherapy and has potent, synergistic BP-lowering effects when combined with other antihypertensive agents, particularly those that block the RAAS. Diuretics also reduce HTN-related morbidity and mortality. Many physicians consider thiazides the diuretics of choice for long-term BP control. Additionally, JNC 7 guidelines recommend including a thiazide diuretic in the initial management of essential HTN.[10] However, not all agree that these agents are preferred over all others; individualization of choices based on medical comorbidity and tolerability is the main consideration.

Thiazide diuretics are among the best-studied agents for BP reduction, and their beneficial effect on the reduction of HTN-related morbidity and mortality is unquestionable. In the Antihypertensive and Lipid-Lowering Treatment to Prevent Heart Attack Trial (ALLHAT), monotherapy with thiazide therapy was associated with no statistically significant differences in the composite primary endpoints of fatal coronary heart disease or nonfatal MI compared to lisinopril and amlodipine; however, thiazide therapy was superior with respect to reducing heart failure (vs. amlodipine and lisinopril) and stroke (vs. lisinopril).[11] Less BP reduction and more CV outcomes were especially evident in blacks treated with ACE inhibitor monotherapy. These results solidified the role of thiazide diuretics in the armament of antihypertensive agents, particularly as a first-line agent.

Low-dose diuretic therapies are generally well tolerated and have been shown to not impair quality of life. Thiazides can increase potassium and magnesium excretion, potentially leading to hypokalemia and hypomagnesemia. Hypokalemia may be responsible for thiazide-related dysglycemia. To date, no analyses of ALLHAT data have indicated that the development of diabetes nullifies the antihypertensive benefit of thiazides. Thiazides can increase serum lipid levels, primarily total cholesterol and low-density lipoprotein cholesterol levels, by approximately 5% to 7% in the first year of therapy. Thiazides are generally considered ineffective when the glomerular filtration rate is less than 30 to 40 mL/min/1.73 m^2, and under these circumstances a loop diuretic should generally be substituted if a volume component is suspected to contribute to the hypertensive process.

Thiazide diuretics, among the least expensive antihypertensive drugs, are also among the most effective for patients with a low-renin and salt-sensitive physiology. This is characteristic of HTN in African-American and older populations. With proper attention to appropriate selection, dosing, and monitoring, diuretic-based regimens can greatly improve the ability to achieve BP goals.

Calcium-Channel Blockers

Long-acting calcium-channel blockers (CCBs) are effective BP-lowering agents that can be used as monotherapy or in combination with diuretics or RAAS blockers for the treatment of essential HTN. One of the best-studied CCBs is the long-acting dihydropyridine amlodipine. The benefits of amlodipine may transcend mere BP reduction. In the Comparison of Amlodipine vs. Enalapril to Limit Occurrences of Thrombosis (CAMELOT) study, the administration of amlodipine to patients with coronary artery disease (CAD) and normal BP resulted in reduced adverse CV events similar to the enalapril group, despite no statistically significant difference in BP reduction between the two groups.[12] Also, amlodipine use was associated with slower atherosclerosis progression by intravascular ultrasound than enalapril.[12] In the Prospective Randomized Evaluation of the Vascular Effects of Norvasc Trial (PREVENT), amlodipine was associated with fewer hospitalizations for unstable angina and revascularization in individuals with CAD, although no change in major CV event rates was recognized.[13] As will be discussed later, when amlodipine was combined with an ACE inhibitor in the Avoiding Cardiovascular Events through Combination Therapy in Patients Living with Systolic HTN (ACCOMPLISH) study, there were fewer CV and renal events compared with patients being treated with a thiazide diuretic and an ACE inhibitor.

Tolerability may be a concern with dihydropyridine CCBs given their propensity to cause lower-extremity edema. This may be of particular concern in younger, female patients or people who are overweight. On the other hand, CCBs may be better suited for older, male patients because they do not affect libido like diuretics and beta-blockers. CCBs may be more effective as monotherapy for BP reduction than RAAS blockers in older and African-American patients. In general, CCBs are effective in reducing BP regardless of age, gender, ethnicity, salt intake, and even concomitant use of nonsteroidal anti-inflammatory drugs.

Beta-Blockers

The administration of beta-blockers to individuals with MI and/or congestive heart failure is a powerful strategy to reduce future CV events and is well supported by the medical literature. To date, however, there is no evidence supporting beta-blockade as an effective method for primary prevention of CV events. Conversely, beta-blockade in hypertensive individuals without compelling CV indications may result in more CV events (particularly strokes) than individuals treated with other types of antihypertensive agents.[14] Beta-blockers are generally well tolerated in clinical practice, although dose-dependent side effects (fatigue, depression, impaired exercise tolerance, and sexual dysfunction) may limit their widespread use. Newer beta-blockers, particularly agents with vasodilatory properties, may have better side-effect profiles than traditional beta-blockers. Large, prospective HTN outcome trials, particularly to evaluate primary prevention of CV outcomes, are necessary before using the newer beta-blockers as first-line therapy for HTN.

Combination Therapy

The optimal combination drug therapy for HTN is not established, although current U.S. guidelines recommend inclusion of a diuretic. The recent ACCOMPLISH trial determined that combination therapy with an ACE inhibitor (benazepril) and a CCB (amlodipine) was superior to the benazepril–hydrochlorothiazide combination in reducing CV and renal events in patients with HTN (>20 mm Hg/10 mm Hg above goal) who were at high risk for CV events.[15,16] The difference in CV event reduction rates occurred despite similar degrees of BP reduction in both combination groups. Based on this study, ACE inhibitors and CCBs may be more appropriate agents for the treatment of HTN in order to allow maximum CV and renal risk reduction when combination therapy (ACE inhibitor and CCB) is necessary.

The combination of various forms of RAAS-blocking agents with other drugs has proven valuable in reducing CV events in individuals with proteinuric kidney disease and congestive heart failure. However, based on the Ongoing Telmisartan Alone and in Combination with Ramipril Global Endpoint Trial (ONTARGET), dual RAAS blockade should be avoided for the management of non-proteinuric, uncomplicated essential HTN given the risk of more adverse events without an increase in CV benefit.[8]

Other Vasodilating Agents

Hydralazine

Hydralazine is a direct smooth muscle relaxant that reduces systemic vascular resistance and thus systemic arterial pressure. Hydralazine is generally not considered a first-line BP medication, primarily because it can induce a reflex tachycardia that can increase myocardial oxygen demands, resulting in ischemia. Hydralazine can also induce marked fluid retention. Its use is generally reserved for refractory HTN or the treatment of pregnancy-related HTN.

Minoxidil

Minoxidil is a potent vasodilator that can be used for the treatment of severe HTN. Like most vasodilators, minoxidil is associated with reflex tachycardia and fluid retention, and concomitant use of a beta-blocker and a loop diuretic is generally necessary. Minoxidil has serious, unfavorable side effects that mandate close monitoring, including hypertrichosis, breast tenderness, and pericarditis. Minoxidil should be reserved for the treatment of severe, refractory HTN.

Alpha-Blockers

The ALLHAT study demonstrated that the lesser BP reduction associated with doxazosin monotherapy was associated with a significantly increased risk of heart failure compared to both chlorthalidone and ACE inhibitors, in addition to a higher rate of overall CV events.[11] Thus, alpha-blockers are not recommended for initial monotherapy, with the possible exception of older men with symptoms of benign prostatic hypertrophy (BPH), particularly if they are at low CV risk.

Sympatholytics

Centrally acting agents are effective antihypertensive agents but have a higher incidence of dose-dependent side effects and lack CV outcome data. Clonidine, a direct alpha-2 agonist, is the most commonly used sympatholytic in clinical practice. It has the advantage of both oral and transdermal administration. Unfortunately, adverse effects, including dry mouth and fatigue, are relatively common. Also, the sudden discontinuation of clonidine can cause rebound HTN due to an abrupt restoration of sympathetic outflow. As a consequence, discontinuation of the medication must be performed in a tapered fashion.

Agents for Resistant HTN

Mineralocorticoid Receptor Antagonists

Aldosterone receptor antagonists are effective adjuncts to traditional antihypertensive regimens. Spironolactone has demonstrated effectiveness in lowering BP in resistant HTN (i.e., BP treatment requiring three or more drugs).[17] Spironolactone use may be limited by adverse effects, including breast tenderness, gynecomastia, loss of libido, and hyperkalemia. Eplerenone is more specific for the mineralocorticoid receptor than spironolactone and as a result has a low occurrence of breast tenderness, gynecomastia, and sexual dysfunction. Mineralocorticoid receptor antagonists have proven effective in the treatment of congestive heart failure, reducing proteinuria, and cirrhosis-related edema. The CV protective effect of mineralocorticoid receptor antagonists in individuals with essential HTN has not been studied.

Potassium-Sparing Diuretics

The benefit of amiloride as adjunct therapy in treating resistant HTN has been demonstrated in observational studies. By blocking the epithelial sodium channel (ENaC), amiloride acts as an indirect aldosterone antagonist since aldosterone induces sodium and fluid retention, in part through upregulation of ENaC. The addition of amiloride to existing multidrug regimens in patients with resistant HTN results in further BP reduction, even when combined with other diuretics. Amiloride is generally less expensive and more tolerable than mineralocorticoid receptor antagonists and therefore should be considered an option for the management of resistant HTN. Amiloride is also available in combination formulations, together with aliskiren (Tekamlo) and with aliskiren and hydrochlorothiazide (Amturinide).

Special Scenarios

Diabetes

The optimal target for BP control in patients with diabetes mellitus remains elusive. The recent Action to Control Cardiovascular Risk in Diabetes Blood Pressure (ACCORD BP) trial showed no reduction in the rate of a composite outcome of fatal and nonfatal major CV events in patients with type 2 diabetes treated to a target SBP of less than 120 mm Hg, compared to standard-therapy group, treated to a target SBP of less than 140 mm Hg.[18] However, both arms achieved excellent BP control: 133 mm Hg in the standard-control arm versus 119 mm Hg in the intensive-control arm. Also, the intensive-control group had an increased relative risk of serious adverse events compared to the standard-therapy group.[18] It may be more difficult to detect differences between lower levels of BP on CV outcomes even in diabetics. The American Diabetes Association (ADA) currently recommends a target BP of below 130/80 mm Hg in patients with diabetes.[19] In hypertensive, diabetic patients with microalbuminuria or clinical albuminuria, ACE inhibitors or ARBs are strongly recommended.[19]

Coronary Artery Disease

The management of HTN in patients with chronic CAD and chronic stable angina is directed toward preventing primary or secondary CV disease events. For the primary prevention of CAD in HTN, the American Heart Association (AHA) guidelines recommend targeting a BP of below 130/80 mm Hg in individuals with demonstrated CAD or with CAD risk equivalents.[20] The AHA guidelines recommend beta-blockers be considered the drugs of first choice for the treatment of HTN in patients with CAD and angina and for secondary prevention for at least 6 months in the post-MI patient.[20] Patients with HTN and chronic stable angina should be treated with a regimen that includes a beta-blocker in patients with a history of prior MI, an ACE inhibitor or ARB if there is diabetes mellitus and/or LV systolic dysfunction, and a thiazide diuretic.[20] If either the angina or the HTN remains uncontrolled, a long-acting dihydropyridine CCB can be added to the regimen.[20]

Chronic Kidney Disease

The goals of antihypertensive therapy in patients with chronic kidney disease (CKD) are to lower BP, reduce the risk of CV disease, and slow progression of CKD. The National Kidney Foundation (NKF) K/DOQI guidelines recommend a target BP of less than 130/80 mm Hg in individuals with CKD, regardless of the cause.[21] ACE inhibitors or ARBs are the preferred therapy for the treatment of HTN in individuals with diabetic nephropathy or non-diabetic kidney disease with a spot protein-to-creatinine ratio of 200 mg/g or higher.[21] Therapy with ACE inhibitors or ARBs, as a method of slowing CKD progression in non-proteinuric CKD patients, is less well defined.

Conclusion

BP control remains the cornerstone of primary CV disease prevention. BP treatment is complex, owing to population diversity, various phenotypic/genotypic expressions of the disease process, and numerous confounding factors to BP control. BP-reduction strategies require a global assessment of multiple factors, including age, sex, ethnicity, and environmental factors. Short of compelling indications for specific BP agents, antihypertensive agents should be selected based on their tolerability and efficacy profiles. Good tolerability, low cost, and simplicity of drug regimen will improve long-term adherence to prescribed antihypertensive regimens. Given the dynamic nature of BP management, clinical inertia on the part of physicians must be avoided to ensure long-term success.

Acknowledgment

We thank Tia A. Paul, University of Maryland School of Medicine, Baltimore, MD, for expert secretarial support.

References

1. Appel LJ, Moore TJ, Obarzanek E, et al. A clinical trial of the effects of dietary patterns on blood pressure. DASH Collaborative Research Group. *N Engl J Med* 1997;336:1117–1124.

2. Sacks FM, Svetkey LP, Vollmer WM, et al. Effects on blood pressure of reduced dietary sodium and the Dietary Approaches to Stop Hypertension (DASH) diet. DASH-Sodium Collaborative Research Group. *N Engl J Med* 2001;344:3–10.

3. Cook NR, Cutler JA, Obarzanek E, et al. Long term effects of dietary sodium reduction on cardiovascular disease outcomes: observational follow-up of the Trials of Hypertension Prevention (TOHP). *BMJ* 2007;334:885–888.

4. Fang J, Wylie-Rosett J, Alderman MH. Exercise and cardiovascular outcomes by hypertensive status: NHANES I epidemiological follow-up study, 1971–1992. *Am J Hypertens* 2005;18:751–758.

5. Yusuf S, Sleight P, Pogue J, et al. Effects of an angiotensin-converting-enzyme inhibitor, ramipril, on cardiovascular events in high-risk patients. The Heart Outcomes Prevention Evaluation Study Investigators. *N Engl J Med* 2000;342:145–153.

6. Dahlof B, Devereux RB, Kjeldsen SE, et al. Cardiovascular morbidity and mortality in the Losartan Intervention For Endpoint reduction in hypertension study (LIFE): a randomised trial against atenolol. *Lancet* 2002;359:995–1003.

7. Lithell H, Hansson L, Skoog I, et al. The Study on Cognition and Prognosis in the Elderly (SCOPE): principal results of a randomized double-blind intervention trial. *J Hypertens* 2003;21:875–886.

8. Yusuf S, Teo KK, Pogue J, et al. Telmisartan, ramipril, or both in patients at high risk for vascular events. *N Engl J Med* 2008;358:1547–1559.

9. Parving HH, Persson F, Lewis JB, et al. Aliskiren combined with losartan in type 2 diabetes and nephropathy. *N Engl J Med* 2008;358:2433–2446.

10. Chobanian AV, Bakris GL, Black HR, et al. Seventh report of the Joint National Committee on Prevention, Detection, Evaluation, and Treatment of High Blood Pressure. *Hypertension* 2003;42:1206–1252.

11. Major outcomes in high-risk hypertensive patients randomized to angiotensin-converting enzyme inhibitor or calcium channel blocker vs. diuretic: The Antihypertensive and Lipid-Lowering Treatment to Prevent Heart Attack Trial (ALLHAT). *JAMA* 2002;288:2981–2997.

12. Nissen SE, Tuzcu EM, Libby P, et al. Effect of antihypertensive agents on cardiovascular events in patients with coronary disease and normal blood pressure: the CAMELOT study: a randomized controlled trial. *JAMA* 2004;292:2217–2225.

13. Pitt B, Byington RP, Furberg CD, et al. Effect of amlodipine on the progression of atherosclerosis and the occurrence of clinical events. PREVENT Investigators. *Circulation* 2000;102:1503–1510.

14. Lindholm LH, Carlberg B, Samuelsson O. Should beta blockers remain first choice in the treatment of primary hypertension? A meta-analysis. *Lancet* 2005;366:1545–1553.

15. Jamerson K, Weber MA, Bakris GL, et al. Benazepril plus amlodipine or hydrochlorothiazide for hypertension in high-risk patients. *N Engl J Med* 2008;359:2417–2428.

16. Bakris GL, Sarafidis PA, Weir MR, et al. Renal outcomes with different fixed-dose combination therapies in patients with hypertension at high risk for cardiovascular events (ACCOMPLISH): a prespecified secondary analysis of a randomised controlled trial. *Lancet* 2010;375:1173–1181.

17. Nishizaka MK, Zaman MA, Calhoun DA. Efficacy of low-dose spironolactone in subjects with resistant hypertension. *Am J Hypertens* 2003;16:925–930.

18. Effects of intensive blood-pressure control in type 2 diabetes mellitus. *N Engl J Med* 2010;362:1575–1585.

19. Arauz-Pacheco C, Parrott MA, Raskin P. The treatment of hypertension in adult patients with diabetes. *Diabetes Care* 2002;25:134–147.

20. Rosendorff C, Black HR, Cannon CP, et al. Treatment of hypertension in the prevention and management of ischemic heart disease: a scientific statement from the American Heart Association Council for High Blood Pressure Research and the Councils on Clinical Cardiology and Epidemiology and Prevention. *Circulation* 2007;115:2761–2788.

21. K/DOQI clinical practice guidelines on hypertension and antihypertensive agents in chronic kidney disease, *Am J Kidney Dis* 2004;43:S1–290.

Chapter 5

Managing Comorbidities

a. Ischemic Heart Disease

Matthew J. Sorrentino, MD

> A 54-year-old African-American man comes to the office for consultation about his elevated BP. He has known CAD and suffered a small MI involving the inferior wall of the left ventricle 5 years previously. He continues to have mild angina pectoris with exertion that is relieved by rest and is thought to be stable. Overall cardiac function remains preserved with an ejection fraction by echocardiography of 54%. His medications include atenolol 25 mg daily and aspirin 81 mg daily. He has no allergies.
>
> On exam in the office his BP is 160/98 mm Hg and his heart rate is 60 bpm. His exam shows signs of fluid retention with a mild elevation in his jugular venous pulsation and 1+ ankle edema. Heart sou\nds are normal with the exception of a fourth heart sound.

The management of HTN in patients with known coronary heart disease should focus on the prevention of CV events and the reduction of myocardial ischemia and relief of symptoms. JNC 7 recommended treating systolic and diastolic BP to less than 140/90 mm Hg except in individuals with diabetes or renal disease, where the recommended goal is less than 130/80 mm Hg.[1] An American Heart Association (AHA) Scientific Statement published in 2007 recommended a BP target of less than 130/80 for patients with demonstrated coronary artery disease (CAD) or CAD risk-equivalent disease, defined as patients with carotid artery disease, peripheral artery disease, or an abdominal aortic aneurysm, or patients with a high risk Framingham risk score.[2] In addition, the statement recommended considering lowering the BP goal to less than 120/80 in patients with heart failure.

The AHA BP recommendations for patients with CAD were based in part on the results of the CAMELOT (Comparison of Amlodipine vs Enalapril to Limit Occurrences of Thrombosis) study.[3] This study was a double-blind, randomized trial comparing amlodipine or enalapril with placebo on CV events in patients with angiographically documented CAD and normal BP. BP averaged 129/78 for all patients and decreased approximately 5/2.5 mm Hg in the treatment groups. CV events were significantly reduced in the amlodipine group, with similar but not significant effects observed in the enalapril group. This suggests that high-risk patients with target organ disease such as CAD may obtain benefit from BP lowering when resting BPs are at what have been traditionally accepted as normal levels.

There remains some concern, however, that excessive lowering of DBP may impair coronary artery perfusion and cause ischemia, leading to an increase in CV events. Studies attempting to demonstrate the presence of a U-shaped or

J-shaped relationship between further DBP lowering and an increase in events are inconclusive. Large epidemiologic studies have shown a linear association between increasing DBP and CV disease risk beginning at 75 mm Hg.[4] A meta-analysis of seven randomized clinical trials observed a J-shaped relationship between DBP and mortality in both treated and untreated subjects and concluded that the increased risk was not a BP treatment effect.[5] Patients with the lowest DBPs or the widest pulse pressures may represent a less healthy cohort. Since some uncertainty remains about the potential for increasing ischemia with lowering DBP, it is recommended to lower BP slowly in patients with CAD and to use caution in older hypertensive individuals or patients with diabetes when lowering DBP below 60 mm Hg.[2]

In addition to a therapeutic lifestyle program, the JNC 7 recommends pharmacologic therapy based on compelling indications for certain antihypertensive drugs for high-risk conditions based on favorable outcome data from clinical trials.[1]

Beta-Blockers

Beta-blockers are the drugs of first choice for patients with HTN and chronic stable angina. Beta-blockers reduce ischemia and angina by reducing heart rate and negative inotropic effects. Beta-blockers with intrinsic sympathomimetic activity (pindolol and acebutolol) should be avoided. Cardioselective beta-blockers are most frequently used, although nonselective beta-blockers have been shown to be effective. A number of investigators have recently questioned the value of beta-blockers and of atenolol in particular in the primary prevention of CV events in hypertensive patients.[6] These concerns, however, likely do not apply to secondary prevention patients since randomized studies in patients with CAD have clearly demonstrated clinical benefits.

Beta-blockers are indicated in patients after an MI and heart failure patients. For hypertensive patients presenting with an acute coronary syndrome, beta-blockers are recommended intravenously at the time of presentation and then orally once the patient is stable. Beta-blockers should be continued indefinitely in patients after an MI. For patients with heart failure, the beta-blockers carvedilol, metoprolol succinate, and bisoprolol have been shown to improve outcomes. Beta-blockers are relatively contraindicated in patients with advanced conduction system disease and active bronchospasm.

Calcium-Channel Blockers

Calcium-channel blockers (CCBs) reduce myocardial oxygen demand and vasodilate coronary arteries and are therefore indicated in the treatment of chronic stable angina and ischemic heart disease. In addition, the nondihydropyridine CCBs diltiazem and verapamil slow the sinus heart rate and decrease conduction through the AV node. CCBs can be used in combination with beta-blockers to further reduce BP or alleviate angina. Long-acting dihydropyridine CCBs are preferred over non-dihydropyridine CCBs when used in combination with beta-blockers to avoid excessive bradycardia. CCBs are recommended as a substitute for beta-blockers in patients who have a contraindication to beta-blockers such as active bronchospasm. CCBs can also relieve angina in patients with vasospastic angina. Short-acting agents should be avoided. The non-dihydropyridine CCBs should not be used in patients with left ventricular dysfunction.

Angiotensin-Converting Enzyme (ACE) Inhibitors and Angiotensin Receptor Blockers (ARBs)

ACE inhibitors are indicated for patients with diabetes and heart failure and are recommended for all patients after an MI. ACE inhibitors are also of benefit in patients with chronic CAD. Several studies, such as the Heart Outcomes Prevention Evaluation (HOPE) study[7] and the European Trial on Reduction of Cardiac Events with Perindopril in Stable Coronary Artery Disease (EUROPA) study,[8] have shown reductions in CV events in individuals with established CAD or at high risk for the development of CV disease with the use of ACE inhibitors compared with placebo. This benefit was observed in patients with and without HTN at baseline. ARBs are generally used in patients who are intolerant of ACE inhibitors.

Diuretics

Thiazide-type diuretics are highly effective BP-lowering agents and are especially useful in patients who present with signs of volume overload. In primary prevention trials such as the Antihypertensive and Lipid-Lowering Treatment to Prevent Heart Attack Trial (ALLHAT), a thiazide diuretic was found to be equivalent to an ACE inhibitor and CCB for CV event reduction.[9] There has been some concern that thiazides may worsen glycemic control, but this effect may be mediated by combined use with an ACE inhibitor or ARB. Aldosterone antagonists such as spironolactone and eplerenone lower BP and are indicated in patients with severe heart failure or after an MI.

Treatment

The patient presented above has chronic angina, a previous MI, and signs of fluid retention. He has an indication for a beta-blocker since he is post MI and has angina. We would recommend a long-acting selective beta-blocker such as metoprolol succinate, targeting his resting heart rate to between 50 and 60 bpm. Since he continues to have angina, the addition of a long-acting dihydropyridine CCB such as amlodipine may help further reduce his angina. He has signs of volume overload, which can be treated with a thiazide diuretic to obtain further BP control and euvolemia. Alternatively, since he has CAD and he is post MI, an ACE inhibitor is indicated and the further reduction in BP may help reduce his angina. His BP goal according to the AHA statement is less than 130/80 mm Hg.

References

1. Chobanian AV, Bakris GL, Black HR, et al. The Seventh Report of the Joint National Committee on Prevention, Detection, Evaluation, and Treatment of High Blood Pressure: the JNC 7 report. *JAMA* 2003;289(19):2560–2572.

2. Rosendorff C, Black HR, Cannon CP, et al. Treatment of hypertension in the prevention and management of ischemic heart disease: a scientific statement from the American Heart Association Council for High Blood Pressure Research and the Councils on Clinical Cardiology and Epidemiology and Prevention. *Circulation* 2007;115(21):2761–2788.

3. Nissen SE, Tuzcu EM, Libby P, et al. Effect of antihypertensive agents on cardiovascular events in patients with coronary disease and normal blood pressure: the CAMELOT study: a randomized controlled trial. *JAMA* 2004;292(18):2217–2225.

4. Lewington S, Clarke R, Qizilbash N, Peto R, Collins R. Age-specific relevance of usual blood pressure to vascular mortality: a meta-analysis of individual data for one million adults in 61 prospective studies. *Lancet* 2002;360(9349):1903–1913.

5. Boutitie F, Gueyffier F, Pocock S, Fagard R, Boissel JP. J-shaped relationship between blood pressure and mortality in hypertensive patients: new insights from a meta-analysis of individual-patient data. *Ann Intern Med* 2002;136(6):438–448.

6. Ong HT. Beta blockers in hypertension and cardiovascular disease. *BMJ* 2007;334(7600):946–949.

7. Yusuf S, Sleight P, Pogue J, Bosch J, Davies R, Dagenais G. Effects of an angiotensin-converting-enzyme inhibitor, ramipril, on cardiovascular events in high-risk patients. The Heart Outcomes Prevention Evaluation Study Investigators. *N Engl J Med* 2000;342(3):145–153.

8. Fox KM. Efficacy of perindopril in reduction of cardiovascular events among patients with stable coronary artery disease: randomised, double-blind, placebo-controlled, multicentre trial (the EUROPA study). *Lancet* 2003;362(9386):782–788.

9. Major outcomes in high-risk hypertensive patients randomized to angiotensin-converting enzyme inhibitor or calcium channel blocker vs. diuretic: The Antihypertensive and Lipid-Lowering Treatment to Prevent Heart Attack Trial (ALLHAT). *JAMA* 2002;288(23):2981–2997.

b. Heart Failure

Melissa Gunasekera, MD and John D. Bisognano, MD, PhD

A wide variety of CV insults may cause congestive heart failure. HTN places an increased afterload strain against through various mechanisms, including sodium and water retention, reduced vascular compliance, arteriolar vasoconstriction, and activation of neurohormonal systems. In response to these mechanisms, the left ventricle hypertrophies in a concentric manner to compensate, causing a longer isovolumic relaxation time and reduced diastolic compliance with diastolic dysfunction. Later in the course of systemic hypertension, increased LV mass may be insufficient to maintain high wall tension caused by elevated pressures, demonstrated by a reduction in contractile capacity resulting in systolic dysfunction.

The worldwide burden of heart failure is great—20 million people—and it is an increasingly common cause of morbidity and mortality.[1] The most prevalent risk factors for heart failure include older age, ischemic heart disease, HTN, and obesity, which may predispose to other conditions such as anemia, diabetes, depression, and sleep apnea, a condition that can further worsen HTN and cardiac function. Both CV and non-CV comorbid conditions are present in patients with heart failure; patients often have three or more significant comorbid conditions. Comorbidities in heart failure may contribute to the cause of the disease as well as have a role in progression and response to therapy. The increased burden of comorbidity in heart failure is associated with an increased hospitalization rate, increased hospital length of stay, and increased mortality.[2] This part of the chapter will address various heart failure comorbidities, including CAD, obesity, diabetes mellitus, anemia, and renal failure. Although heart failure, in itself, is a formidable disease, it is also important to recognize that most patients with heart failure have other associated problems.

Coronary Artery Disease

CAD remains the most common identifiable process underlying heart failure in the United States, and HTN is an important contributor to the risk of CAD. The impairment of systolic and diastolic dysfunction is often seen in patients with heart failure due to CAD. This is secondary to compromised sub-endocardial perfusion causing elevations in LV diastolic pressures, which diminish the diastolic trans-coronary perfusion gradient. Primary pump dysfunction leads to activation of multiple neurohormonal mechanisms that adversely load the failing heart. The reported prevalence of CAD in patients with heart failure ranges widely. Choudhury et al. reviewed the relationship between CAD, ischemia, and heart failure, noting that chronic CAD can induce both impaired relaxation as well as increased diastolic stiffness.[3] In the ADHERE database with over 100,000 heart failure admissions, 55% of patients have evidence of CAD.[4] Franciosa et al. followed 182 patients with chronic heart failure and reported 2-year mortality rates of 69% in patients with CAD versus 48% in those with idiopathic dilated cardiomyopathy.[5] In a series of 860 patients with known or suspected CAD evaluated at the Mayo Clinic, Chuah et al. reported that a history of heart failure was the most important clinical predictor of cardiac events.[6]

Diabetes Mellitus

Diabetes mellitus is found in approximately one quarter of outpatients with heart failure and almost half of patients hospitalized for heart failure.[7] The Framingham Heart Study found that diabetic men had a twofold elevated risk of developing heart failure, while diabetic women had a fourfold elevated risk.[8] In diabetics with poor glycemic control, the risk of heart failure is magnified: for each 1% increase in the HbA1c level, the risk of heart failure increases by 8%.[9] Other diabetes-related risk factors such as HTN, CAD, and LV hypertrophy all independently contribute to the development of heart failure.

Heart failure itself has been found to increase the risk of insulin resistance and diabetes. Shah et al. found that the risk of diabetes increased with heart failure severity because underlying mechanisms may directly promote the development of insulin resistance in heart failure, including elevating circulating free fatty acids and sympathetic nervous system activation.[10] Cardiotoxic effects of hyperglycemia and insulin resistance include cardiac hypertrophy, endothelial dysfunction, inflammation, and lipotoxicity.[10] Analyses from the Left Ventricular Dysfunction (SOLVD) trial have shown that diabetes is a risk factor for progression from asymptomatic LV dysfunction to symptomatic heart failure, as well as a risk factor for all-cause mortality.[11] The increased mortality risk associated with diabetes has been observed in additional heart failure cohorts, including elderly patients with chronic and new-onset heart failure, as well as advanced heart failure patients in transplant referral centers.[12]

Obesity

Obesity is an increasingly prevalent condition present in approximately one third of the U.S. population.[13] Both increased circulating blood volume and cardiac output are associated with elevated body mass index (BMI). Obesity is associated with multiple CV risk factors with the potential to promote the development of heart failure, including hypertension, LV hypertrophy, CAD, diabetes, and dyslipidemia.[14] In a Framingham study analysis, overweight status (defined as BMI >25 kg/m^2) conferred a 34% increased risk of developing heart failure, while obesity (defined as BMI >30 kg/m^2) conferred a 104% increased risk.

However, once heart failure has been established, epidemiology reverses, as several studies have demonstrated that elevated BMI is not associated with increased risk in chronic heart failure and instead confers an improved prognosis.[15] The pathophysiology behind this paradoxical relationship is incompletely understood, though current theories propose that obese patients may have an increased metabolic reserve and less cytokine activation. Cardiac cachexia is an independent predictor of poor heart failure outcomes, reflecting a state of sympathetic activation and catabolic imbalance.[16]

Renal Failure

Recently, renal dysfunction has been recognized as an important predictor of morbidity and mortality due to heart failure. A low glomerular filtration rate (GFR) of less than 60 mL/min in heart failure patients is thought to be a consequence of diminished cardiac output, with decreased renal perfusion and intrarenal vasoconstriction. This is accompanied by sodium and water retention, causing an impaired escape from aldosterone and resistance to natriuretic peptides. There are many potential mechanisms whereby renal dysfunction may contribute to the progression of heart failure, such as increased myocardial remodeling causing LV dilatation and resultant worsening mitral regurgitation, leading to increased LV wall mass and increased myocardial fibrosis with myocyte apoptosis.[17]

The increased risk of mortality conferred by renal dysfunction was found to be as important as other prognostic factors such as NYHA functional classification, age, LV ejection fraction, and diabetes.[18] In the Studies of Left Ventricular Dysfunction (SOLVD), a GFR of less than 60 mL/min was noted in 21% of subjects in the prevention trial and 36% in the treatment trial, despite exclusion for a plasma creatinine of more than 2 mg/dL.[18] In both the prevention and treatment arms of the SOLVD studies, worsening renal failure was primarily predictive for an increase in pump failure deaths and hospitalizations for heart failure, with little predictive value for arrhythmic death.[18] This has led to the speculation that renal dysfunction may be not only a marker for worsening heart failure but also a factor exacerbating the progression of heart failure. Worsening renal failure in patients with decompensated heart failure is a potent predictor of mortality. In a prospective cohort of 412 patients hospitalized for heart failure, a plasma creatinine elevation of 0.1 mg/dL or more and more than 0.5 mg/dL occurred in 75% and 24% of patients, respectively, where mortality was increased in patients with greater elevations in plasma creatinine.[19]

Anemia

Anemia has been recognized as a common condition in patients with heart failure, with a prevalence ranging from 4% to 55%.[20] Interestingly, the prevalence of anemia increases with severity of heart failure, as seen by the presence of anemia in 4% of patients with mild to moderate heart failure compared to 49% of patients with acute decompensated heart failure.[20] Heart failure with anemia is associated with increased severity of disease as lower hemoglobin levels have correlated with higher NYHA class, lower exercise capacity, decreased LV ejection fraction, an impaired hemodynamic profile, as well as increased B-type natriuretic peptide and cardiac troponin levels.[21] In the Framingham study, lower hematocrit was associated with an increased risk of developing heart failure, and anemia in end-stage renal disease has been associated with increased heart failure.[22] Anemia may be a marker of a disease severity, reflecting any combination of factors, including inflammatory cytokine activation, volume overload, renal insufficiency, malnutrition, or increased burden of medical comorbidities. The association of anemia with adverse clinical outcomes in heart failure has led to interest in anemia as a potential therapeutic target; the use of recombinant erythropoietin to treat anemia in heart failure patients has been explored in small studies with promising results.[23]

The treatment of systolic heart failure is multifaceted, and goals include alleviating symptoms, reducing hospitalizations, and slowing progressive LV remodeling. Several clinical trials have studied the use of ACE inhibitors, including the Studies of Left Ventricular Dysfunction (SOLVD), the Acute Infarction Ramipril Efficacy Study (AIRE), and the Heart Outcomes Protection Evaluation (HOPE), and have indicated a reduction in LV remodeling and a decreased occurrence of heart failure among high-risk patients. Angiotensin receptor blockers (ARBs) should be given to patients who cannot tolerate ACE inhibitors, as several studies show ARBs to be superior to placebo, including the Candesartan in Heart Failure Assessment of Reduction in Morbidity and Mortality (CHARM) trial. The treatment of systolic dysfunction with beta-blocker therapy has been shown to decrease mortality, with reductions in heart rate and BP, and to exert beneficial anti-ischemic effects. The Randomized Aldosterone Evaluation Study (RALES) with spironolactone demonstrated a decrease in mortality in heart failure patients. Implantable cardioverter-defibrillator (ICD) placement should be considered as prophylaxis against arrhythmias in patients with LV ejection fraction below 30%. Despite optimal medical therapy, some patients may advance to severe heart failure with LV systolic dysfunction, and those with a wide QRS should be considered for biventricular pacing. The surgical insertion of assist devices and cardiac transplantation are recommended in patients with severe heart failure, refractory debilitating angina, and ventricular arrhythmias.

The treatment of diastolic heart failure, common in elderly patients with a history of HTN, should target reduction of symptoms, HTN management, and treatment for CAD. Symptom reduction by decreasing pulmonary venous pressure at rest and during exertion using both non-pharmacologic and pharmacologic approaches includes improvement of exercise tolerance, reduction of LV volume with diuretic therapy, and decreasing central blood volume with nitrates. Diuretics and nitrates should be initiated at low doses to avoid hypotension and fatigue, which may be limiting side effects. The use of ACE inhibitors, ARBs, and aldosterone antagonists may improve symptoms due to hypertrophy associated with activation of neurohumoral systems. Beta-blockers and some calcium-channel blockers can be used to prevent tachycardia and control hypertension. Diastolic heart failure caused by pathologic disease such as CAD requires specific therapeutic targets, including treatment of ischemia by increasing myocardial blood flow and reducing myocardial oxygen demand.

Comorbidities in heart failure may both contribute to the cause of the disease and have a key role in its progression as well as response to therapy. Further investigations into medical management of comorbid conditions in heart failure are needed to better treat these patients.

References

1. American Heart Association. Heart disease and stroke statistics—2005 update. http://www.americanheart.org/presenter.jhtml?identifer=3000090. Accessed March 31, 2010.

2. Braunstein JB, Anderson GF, Gerstenblith G, et al. Noncardiac comorbidity increases preventable hospitalizations and mortality among Medicare beneficiaries with chronic heart failure. *J Am Coll Cardiol* 2003;42:1226–1233.

3. Choudhury L, Gherorghiade M, Bonow RO. Coronary artery disease in patients heart failure and preserved systolic function. *Am J Cardiol* 2002;89(6):719–722.

4. Fonarow GC, ADHERE Scientific Advisory Committee. The Acute Decompensated Heart Failure National Registry (ADHERE): opportunities to improve care of patients hospitalized with acute decompensated heart failure. *Rev Cardiovasc Med* 2003;4(Suppl 7):S21–S30.

5. Franciosa JA, Wilen M, Ziesch S, et al. Survival of men with severe chronic left ventricular failure due to either coronary heart disease or idiopathic dilated cardiomyopathy. *Am J Cardiol* 1983;51:831–836.

6. Chuah SC, Pellikka PA, Roger VL, et al. Role of dobutamine stress echocardiography in predicting outcome in 860 patients with known or suspected coronary artery disease. *Circulation* 1998;97:1474–1480.

7. Fonarow GC. The management of the diabetic patient with prior cardiovascular event. *Rev Cardiovasc Med* 2003;4(Suppl 7):S38–S49.

8. Kannel WB. Vital epidemiologic clues in heart failure. *J Clin Epidemiol* 2000;53:229–235.

9. Iribarrren C, Karten AJ, Go AS, et al. Glycemic control and heart failure among adult patients with diabetes. *Circulation* 2001;103:2668–2673.

10. Shah A, Shannon RP. Insulin resistance in dilated cardiomyopathy. *Rev Cardiovasc Med* 2003;4(Suppl 6):S50–S57.

11. Das SR, Drazner MH, Yancy CW, et al. Effects diabetes mellitus and ischemic heart disease on the progression from asymptomatic left ventricular dysfunction to symptomatic heart failure: a retrospective analysis from the Studies of Left Ventricular Dysfunction (SOLVD) Prevention trial. *Am Heart J* 2004;148:883–888.

12. Smooke S, Horwich TB, Fonarow GC. Insulin-treated diabetes is associated with a marked increase in mortality in patients with advanced heart failure. *Am Heart J* 2004;148:883–888.

13. Hedley AA, Ogden CL, Johnson CL, et al. Prevalence of overweight and obesity among US children, adolescents and adults, 1999–2002. *JAMA* 2004;291:2847–2850.

14. Kenchaiah S, Evans JC, Levy D, et al. Obesity and the risk of heart failure. *N Engl J Med* 2002;26(Suppl 4):S15–20.

15. Lavie CJ, Osman, AF, Milani RV, Mehra MR. Body composition and prognosis in chronic systolic heart failure: the obesity paradox. *Am J Cardiol* 2003;91:891–894.

16. Anker SD, Chua TP, Ponikoski P, Varney S, et al. Wasting as independent risk factor for mortality in chronic heart failure. *Lancet* 1997;349:1050–1053.

17. Levy D, Garrison RJ, Savage DD, et al. Prognostic implications of echocardiographically determined left ventricular mass in the Framingham Heart Study. *N Engl J Med* 1990;322(22):1561–1566.

18. Dries DL, Exner DV, Domanski MJ, et al. The prognostic implications of renal insufficiency in asymptomatic and symptomatic patients with left ventricular systolic dysfunction. *J Am Coll Cardiol* 2000;35(3):681–689.

19. Smith KJ, Bleyer AJ, Little WC, et al. The cardiovascular effects erythropoietin. *Cardiovasc Res* 2003;59(3):538–548.

20. Horwich TB, Fonarow GC, Hamilton MA, et al. Anemia is associated with worse symptoms, greater impairment in functional capacity and a significant increase in mortality in patients with advanced heart failure. *J Am Coll Cardiol* 2002;39:1780–1786.

21. Ralli S, Horwich TB, Fonarow GC. Relationship between anemia, cardiac troponin I and B-type natiuretic peptide levels and mortality in patients with advanced heart failure. *Circulation* 2004;110:149–154.

22. Mancini DM, Katz SD, Lang CC, et al. Effect of erythropoietin on exercise capacity in patients with moderate to severe chronic heart failure. *Circulation* 2003;107:294–299.

c. Diabetic Hypertension

Sergio Chang Figueroa, MD, Shadi Barakat, MD, Adam
Whaley-Connell, MD, and James R. Sowers, MD

A 55-year-old man with obesity, hyperlipidemia, and HTN and type 2 diabetes
presents with no specific medical concerns. His current treatment consists of
hydrochlorothiazide, simvastatin, and metformin/glyburide. On physical exam
he is noted to have a seated BP of 152/92 mm Hg and a BMI of 34. There is no
clinical evidence of neuropathy, congestive heart failure, or peripheral vascular
disease. However, he has a serum creatinine of 1.5 mg/dL and microalbuminuria,
with a random first morning void urine protein-to-creatinine ratio of 200 mg/g.
His fasting glucose was 180 mg/dL and HgbA1c was 8.3%.

Prevalent HTN is approximately twice as frequent in patients with type 2 diabetes mellitus compared to those without diabetes, and conversely hypertensive persons are more predisposed to develop type 2 diabetes than normotensive persons.[1,2] Among those with type 1 diabetes, the incidence of HTN rises from 5% at 10 years to 33% at 20 years and 70 percent at 40 years.[3] HTN is one of the leading modifiable risk factors for macrovascular and microvascular complications in diabetic individuals. Indeed, strategies that incorporate reductions in BP, even lowering BP below current treatment thresholds, have been shown over time to reduce the CVD risk in those with type 2 diabetes. Treatment of HTN in the context of type 2 diabetes requires knowledge of its relationship to other metabolic risk factors for CVD and an appropriate comprehension of the CV pathophysiology, available pharmacologic options, and potential adverse effects.[1–3]

Pathogenesis of HTN in Type 2 Diabetes

HTN and insulin resistance are closely interrelated and contribute significantly to CVD and chronic kidney disease (CKD) morbidity and mortality.[1–3] The pathophysiology of HTN involves multiple hereditary and environmental factors. There is increasing evidence that obesity, particularly visceral type, possesses a local renin-angiotensin-aldosterone system (RAAS) and its activity is increased in hyperinsulinemia.[4] Increases in angiotensin II as well as aldosterone have been shown to impair insulin metabolic signaling. This results in reductions in endothelial nitric oxide synthase (eNOS) activation and reductions in bioavailable nitric oxide (NO), with resultant impairment in endothelial-mediated relaxation. Also, hyperinsulinemia/insulin resistance has been shown to promote sodium retention and intravascular volume expansion. Insulin resistance and other associated metabolic abnormalities also promote hypercoagulability, inflammation, and oxidative stress, all of which contribute to the

65

development of microalbuminuria and LV hypertrophy. Microalbuminuria and CKD are components of the metabolic syndrome as well as early markers of CVD. Microalbuminuria is therefore an important predictor of atherosclerosis, progressive CKD, and increased CVD morbidity and mortality.[2]

Complications Related to HTN in Type 2 Diabetes

A strong continuous, graded relationship exists between increasing BP and the risk of CVD and CKD morbidity and mortality. In turn, each incremental reduction in 20 mm Hg SBP or 10 mm Hg DBP is associated with more than a two-fold reduction in stroke, as well as other CVD mortality, without evidence of a threshold down to approximately 115/75 mm Hg.[2] Indeed, the presence of diabetes increases the absolute risk of CVD mortality attributed to HTN even further.[1-3]

Type 2 diabetes and HTN are also the leading causes of CKD and progression to end-stage renal disease (ESRD), and the risk is greater for ESRD attributed to HTN in patients with diabetes than in those without it.[1-3] Similarly, HTN also strongly influences the development of retinopathy as evidenced in the UK Prospective Diabetes Study (UKPDS), where tighter BP control (<150/85 mm Hg vs. <180/105 mm Hg) resulted in a 34% reduction in progression of retinopathy.[5] Finally, diabetic neuropathy worsens with HTN in patients with type 1 diabetes, but the association has not been clearly established in type 2 diabetes.[3,5]

Benefits of Treatment of HTN in Type 2 Diabetes

Current best evidence guideline management recommends a treatment goal for patients with diabetes of below 130/80 mm Hg; however, there is limited clinical evidence to support this recommendation.[1,2] There have been several trials through the years to guide this recommendation, but recent data from the Action to Control Cardiovascular Risk in Diabetes (ACCORD) and Action in Diabetes and Vascular disease: Preterax and Diamicron Modified Release Controlled Evaluation (ADVANCE) studies may challenge this.[6,7]

Early reports from the UKPDS suggested that each 10-mm Hg decrease in SBP leads to significant reductions in risk for any complication related to diabetes, overall mortality related to diabetes, as well as macrovascular and microvascular complications. The mean BP achieved in the UKPDS was 144/82 mm Hg in the more rigorously controlled group (vs. the usual care group, 154/87 mm Hg) and resulted in significant reduction in each of the aforementioned points.[5] Interestingly, on 10-year follow-up the differences in BP were lost within 2 years after cessation of the intervention and the beneficial effects on both macrovascular and microvascular events were not sustained.[8]

Investigators then sought to randomize individuals to an SBP goal of either 120 mm Hg or the more conventional 140 mm Hg in the ACCORD Trial.[6]

Interestingly, after 4.7 years of follow-up there were no differences in the annual rate of the primary outcome (a composite of nonfatal MI, nonfatal stroke, or death from CV causes), with a higher incidence of serious adverse events. Although it is important to note that there was a beneficial effect shown for the secondary endpoint of total stroke, the total number of major coronary disease events was far higher than the number of total strokes. The authors contend that an SBP target below 120 mm Hg in patients with type 2 diabetes is not justified and raises the question of what are appropriate targets in those with diabetes. Similar findings were observed in the ADVANCE study, which compared a combination of perindopril and indapamide versus placebo. There was a significant reduction in macrovascular or microvascular events and mortality in the intensive arm (135/75 mm Hg) compared to the control arm (140/77 mm Hg).[7]

Treatment Recommendations

Any intervention should include lifestyle modifications. This includes following the DASH dietary plan, performing at least 150 minutes of aerobic exercise per week, as well as alcohol moderation and tobacco cessation. Even a modest weight loss, up to 5% to 10% of initial body weight, may reduce the risk of CVD substantially. Pharmacologic therapy should be initiated concomitantly, particularly if BP is above 140/90 mm Hg, in those with diabetes.[1,2]

The JNC 7 recommend that a thiazide-type diuretic be the first medication used in most stage 1 hypertensive patients regardless of the diagnosis of diabetes.[2] However, the American Diabetes Association (ADA) stresses the importance of initial use of either an ACE inhibitor or an ARB, with substantial evidence to support incorporation of inhibitors of the RAAS to prevent incident type 2 diabetes in those with pre-diabetes as well as CVD and CKD endpoints.[1] Nevertheless, the majority of patients with diabetes and HTN will require three or more medications to achieve a SBP of less than 130/80 mm Hg.[1]

ACE inhibitor therapy should be an integral component of any antihypertensive regimen in patients with type 2 diabetes.[1,2] The HOPE trial suggested that the use of an ACE inhibitor reduces rates of death, MI, stroke, revascularization, cardiac arrest, heart failure, and complications related to diabetes independent of the degree of BP reduction. Further data from the Diabetes Reduction Assessment with Ramipril and Rosiglitazone Medication (DREAM) trial as well as the Nateglinide and Valsartan in Impaired Glucose Tolerance Outcomes Research (NAVIGATOR) trial suggest that RAAS inhibition in those who are insulin-resistant reduces the incidence of diabetes. Further preclinical data suggest that the reductions in incident diabetes are likely mediated by improvements in insulin signaling and systemic insulin sensitivity.[4]

The antihypertensive efficacy of ARBs has largely been shown to be equivalent to ACE inhibitors but with an improved side-effect profile, particularly less cough. Similar to ACE inhibitors, ARBs offer additional benefits in patients with type 2 diabetes. Also similar to ACE inhibitors, numerous studies demonstrate significant reductions in the CVD as well as CKD endpoints when incorporating an ARB in the antihypertensive regimen in those with type 2 diabetes.

Thiazide-type diuretics have been the basis of antihypertensive therapy in most outcome trials. In these trials, diuretics have been unsurpassed in preventing the CVD complications of HTN. Diuretics enhance the antihypertensive efficacy of multidrug regimens, are useful in achieving BP control, and are inexpensive. However, they should be used cautiously in patients with gout, hyponatremia, and hypercalcemia. Also, some studies have implicated thiazide diuretics in increasing the incidence of type 2 diabetes. However, there is accumulating evidence that chlorthalidone has beneficial CV outcome effects beyond those of other thiazide diuretics, and this is the preferable agent in diabetic patients with HTN.[9]

When a third medication is needed, a CCB is thought to be a reasonable choice in those with diabetes. The role of CCBs in HTN management in those with type 2 diabetes appears to gain importance in combination strategies, as evidenced in the Avoiding Cardiovascular Events Through Combination Therapy in Patients Living With Systolic Hypertension (ACCOMPLISH) trial, where amlodipine provided better protection against CVD events than low-dose hydrochlorothiazide when both were used in combination with an ACE inhibitor.[10]

Beta-blockers have been implicated in masking of hypoglycemic symptoms and possible exacerbation of peripheral arterial disease and worsening of hyperglycemia. Their role seems to be mainly as an add-on medication, and they have proven effectiveness similar to inhibitors of the RAAS.

Alpha-blockers are effective in patients with type 2 diabetes. However, they are associated with orthostatic hypotension and are not considered first-line treatment but can be added to the BP regimen.

Case Study

Our case introduces the notion that combination therapy is usually necessary to achieve appropriate BP control, especially in those with type 2 diabetes. RAAS inhibition should be initiated upon diagnosis either in combination with a thiazide diuretic or a dihydropyridine CCB; that approach will help prevent deterioration of kidney function and glycemic control. At this point an ACE inhibitor or an ARB should be added; however, a pending discussion should address the appropriate target BP for patients with diabetes. In the current scenario with uncontrolled HTN and microalbuminuria, the JNC 7 recommends targeting a BP less than 130/80 mm Hg. Weight loss and dietary modifications should be made, and secondary causes of HTN, particularly obstructive sleep apnea, should be ruled out.

References

1. Bakris GL, Sowers JR. ASH Position Paper: Treatment of hypertension in patients with diabetes-an update. *J Am Soc Hypertens* 2008;10(9):707–713.

2. Chobanian AV, Bakris GL, Black HR, Cushman WC. The Seventh Report of the Joint National Committee on Prevention, Detection, Evaluation, and Treatment of High Blood Pressure: The JNC 7 Report. *JAMA* 2003;289:2560–2572.

3. Epstein M, Sowers JR. Diabetes mellitus and hypertension. *Hypertension* 1992;19(5):403–418.

4. Sowers JR, Whaley-Connell A, Epstein M. Narrative review: The emerging clinical implications of the role of aldosterone in the metabolic syndrome and resistant hypertension. *Ann Intern Med* 2009;150:776–783.

5. UK Prospective Diabetes Study Group. Tight blood pressure control and risk of macrovascular and microvascular complications in type 2 diabetes: UKPDS 38. *BMJ* 1998;317:703–713.

6. Cushman WC, Evans GW, Byington RP, Goff DC Jr, Grimm RH Jr, Cutler JA, Simons-Morton DG, Basile JN, Corson MA, Probstfield JL, Katz L, Peterson KA, Friedewald WT, Buse JB, Bigger JT, Gerstein HC, Ismail-Beigi F. The ACCORD Study Group. Effects of intensive blood-pressure control in type 2 diabetes mellitus. *N Engl J Med* 2010;362:1575–1585.

7. Patel A; ADVANCE Collaborative Group, MacMahon S, Chalmers J, Neal B, Woodward M, Billot L, Harrap S, Poulter N, Marre M, Cooper M, Glasziou P, Grobbee DE, Hamet P, Heller S, Liu LS, Mancia G, Mogensen CE, Pan CY, Rodgers A, Williams B. Effects of a fixed combination of perindopril and indapamide on macrovascular and microvascular outcomes in patients with type 2 diabetes mellitus (the ADVANCE trial): a randomized controlled trial. *Lancet* 2007;370(9590):829–840.

8. Holman RR, Paul SK, Bethel MA, Neil HAW, Matthews DR. Long-term follow-up after tight control of blood pressure in type 2 diabetes. *N Engl J Med* 2008;359:1565–1576.

9. Kurtz TW. Chlorthalidone: don't call it "thiazide-like" anymore. *Hypertension* 2010 [epub ahead of print].

10. Jamerson K, Weber MA, Bakris GL, Dahlof B, Pitt B, Shi V, Hester A, Gupte J, Gatlin M, Velazquez EJ. Benazepril plus amlodipine or hydrochlorothiazide for hypertension in high-risk patients. *N Engl J Med* 2008;359(23):2417–2428.

d. Chronic Kidney Disease

Victor Marinescu, MD, PhD and
Peter A. McCullough, MD, MPH

Renal Disease and Hypertension

The rising incidence and prevalence of end-stage renal disease (ESRD), compounded with poor outcomes and cost, have made chronic kidney disease (CKD) a worldwide health problem. CKD is defined as an estimated glomerular filtration rate (eGFR) of less than 60 mL/min/1.73 m^2 or the presence of markers of kidney damage for a period of at least 3 months.[1] In the United States, most recent data indicate that the prevalence of CKD has risen to 13.1%,[2] affecting more than 25 million people and leading to ESRD in over 500,000 people (Fig. 5d.1).

HTN has been identified as an independent risk factor in the development of ESRD and in the progression of early kidney disease to ESRD.[3–5] In fact, HTN is second only to diabetes as a leading cause of ESRD in Europe and the United States. This is in part due to the intricate link between the kidney and BP control (or intravascular volume control), a link that involves multiple levels of communication, including the renin-angiotensin system (RAS), sympathetic nervous system (SNS), antidiuretic hormones, endothelin, and natriuretic peptides. In addition, there is genetic predisposition to the development of simultaneous hypertension and CKD.[6] On the other hand, numerous studies have established that chronic parenchymal renal disease is the most common cause of secondary HTN, accounting for approximately 5% of all patients with HTN.[7]

BP Control and Preservation of Renal Function

Mounting evidence from 20- to 30-year follow-ups of older studies as well as more recent clinical trials has shown that the increasing risk of development of CKD/ESRD correlates significantly with rise in BP.[8–13] As an example, an SBP of above 200 mm Hg leads to a 48 times higher risk of ESRD than an SBP of less than 120 mm Hg. Similarly, the percentage of CKD patients with advanced stages of measured HTN increases as CKD stage increases. Subjects with higher BPs had elevated creatinine levels, with values three times higher in those with a DBP of above 115 mm Hg than in those with a DBP of 90 to 114 mm Hg. The Modification of Diet in Renal Disease (MDRD) study has also confirmed a higher incidence of renal failure associated with higher BPs. Most intriguingly,

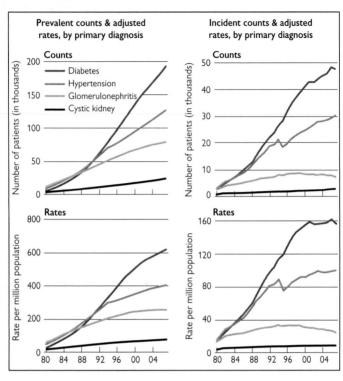

Figure 5d.1 Prevalent and incident counts and adjusted rates of CKD by primary diagnosis. (Adapted from USRDS 2009 Annual Data Report.)

the Physicians' Health Study (PHS) investigated the association between different BP measures and the risk of CKD in apparently healthy men without known kidney disease at baseline. These results showed a clear association between elevated BP and the development of CKD after 14 years of follow-up. Average SBP and pulse pressure (PP) were associated with higher risk for reduced GFR after adjustment for confounding variables, making them strong predictors of reduced GFR of less than 60 mL/min/1.73 m^2 (Fig. 5d.2)[13]

Similar to CVD risk, the relationship between various BP measures and risk of kidney dysfunction can vary by age. While renal excretory function does deteriorate with age beginning in the third or fourth decades of life, this age-related loss of renal function can be significantly accelerated by elevated BP levels. In fact, the rate of GFR deterioration can get as high as 4 to 8 mL/min/year if SBP remains uncontrolled.[14] The elderly are the population most vulnerable to this phenomenon: elevated SBP strongly predicts a decline in kidney function among individuals 70 years of age and up.[15]

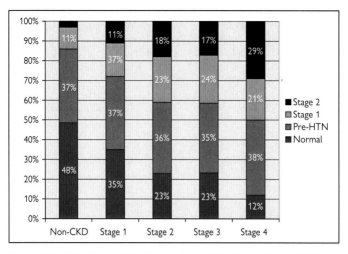

Figure 5d.2 BP classification by CKD stage. (Adapted from Snyder J, Foley R, Collins A. Awareness, treatment, & control of hypertension in chronic kidney disease Stages 1–4 in NHANES 1999–2004 participants. USRDS, Minneapolis Medical Research Foundation, University of Minnesota Twin Cities, 2008.)

Pathophysiology of Systemic HTN in Primary Glomerular Disease

The pathophysiologic mechanisms involved in the progression of CKD with uncontrolled HTN are complex, as glomerular injury activates a variety of pathways that increase arterial BP. These include activation of the SNS and the RAS, sodium retention, volume expansion, and the decreased synthesis of vasodilatory substances such as antidiuretic hormone and natriuretic peptide. Post-mortem studies on kidneys from individuals with essential HTN give us the best clues towards understanding the parallel relationship between HTN and CKD. Measurement of fibroblastic renovasculopathy provides an innovative and accurate way of estimating chronic BP control by using a polynomial regression equation.[16,17]

Prolonged exposure to elevated SBP sets in motion a vicious cycle that causes vasoconstriction, sodium retention, and ultimately renal injury. The inciting event is thought to be increased sympathetic activity[18] or increased release of angiotensin II.[19] Subsequently, kidney dysfunction progresses due to chronic adrenergic exposure, increased levels of endothelin,[20] oxidative stress, and enhanced RAS activity.[21] Glomerular HTN ultimately leads to capillary stretching, endothelial damage, and elevated protein filtration in the kidneys. These processes cause secretion of cytokines, growth factors, and other inflammatory mediators from mesangial cells, which ultimately leads to the replacement of active kidney tissue by connective tissue and fibrosis[22] and a loss of nephrons.[23]

One of the most important factors leading to progression of renal failure appears to be the activation of the RAS, whose consequences are not only BP elevation but also cell proliferation, inflammation, and matrix accumulation.[24–27] This is highlighted by the fact that the renoprotective effects of ACE inhibitors and ARBs are far greater than can be explained by lowering of SBP alone (Fig. 5d.3).[27]

CV Endpoints in Individuals with CKD

Mirroring the trends in the general population, CVD is the number-one cause of death in persons with CKD. In fact, individuals with moderate CKD have an approximately 16% increase in CVD mortality, while those with severe CKD have as much as a 30% increase when compared to the general population.[28] Also, CKD is an independent risk factor for development of resistant HTN, which results in higher mortality rates as well. It comes as no surprise, then, that reduction in BP in patients in CKD has a positive effect on cardiac outcomes and mortality.

Implications in Heart Failure

Cardiomyopathy due to or worsened by pressure and volume overload is the key element that makes heart failure particularly challenging in the set-ting of CKD/ESRD. This is clinically relevant since as many as 20% of patients approaching dialysis carry a diagnosis of heart failure, and the combination of the two leads to higher patient mortality rates (Fig. 5d.4).

The extent to which elevated SBP or DBP contributes to the diagnosis of heart failure in these individuals is still unclear. The greatest challenge to the cardiologist comes from the choice of pharmacologic treatment choices. The clinicians' armamentarium should however include ACE inhibitors, or ARBs if ACE inhibitors are not tolerated, since despite the chronically elevated serum creatinine levels, reduction of intraglomerular pressure does translate to improved survival and reduced rates of ESRD in this patient population. Hyperkalemia and an accelerated course to ESRD should be a concern only once eGFR levels fall below 15 mL/min/1.73 m². In younger individuals, when there is concern about falsely diagnosing CKD due to a creatinine elevation on a RAS blocker, cystatin-C can be used as an alternative marker of renal filtra-tion to follow over time.[29]

Implications in Stroke Prevention

Several studies have specifically examined kidney disease as a risk factor for stroke. Most recently, a secondary analysis of the Bezafibrate Infarction Prevention Trial demonstrated that CKD is an independent risk factor for stroke.[30] Wannamethee et al.[31] examined a cohort of men in the British Regional

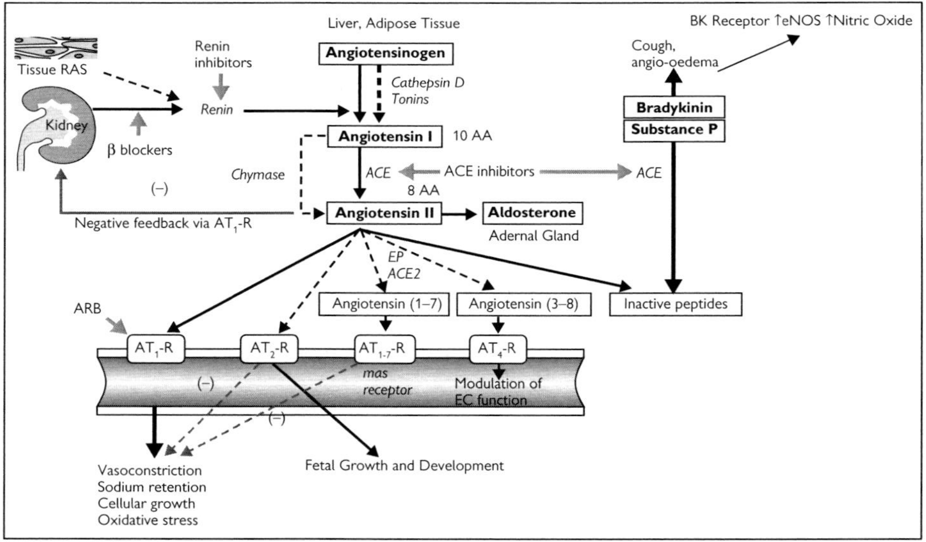

Figure 5d.3 Physiology and pathophysiology of the RAS. (Reprinted with permission from Staessen J, et al. *Lancet North Am Ed* 2006;368:1449–1456.)

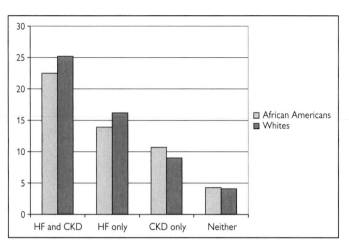

Figure 5d.4 Mortality in patients with CKD, heart failure, or both. (Adapted from USRDS 2008 Annual Data Report.)

Heart Study and found a significantly increased risk for stroke in individuals with the highest 10% of serum creatinine levels. However, neither of these analyses focused on the role of HTN. It has been well documented that HTN is an important risk factor for cerebrovascular disease, with the risk for stroke doubling in the general population with each incremental rise of 20/10 mm Hg above a baseline BP of 115/75 mm Hg.[32] This relationship also holds true for individuals with CKD at elevated BPs, with the only difference being that a J-shaped curve also puts patients with SBP below 110 mm Hg at increased risk for stroke.[33]

Reduction in Coronary Events

While it is clear that tight BP control plays a key role in decreasing CV mortality, mainly by reducing the risk for stroke and heart failure in individuals with CKD, the verdict is not in on CAD. This is mainly because patients with CKD or ESRD have been excluded from the randomized treatment trials from which the algorithms for the prompt diagnosis and treatment of acute coronary syndromes were derived. Retrospective studies have, however, identified CKD as one of the most important prognostic factors for long-term mortality.[34] However, the large ONTARGET trial demonstrated no additional event reduction with a modest reduction in BP when an ARB was added to an ACE inhibitor.[35] In addition, the recent Action to Control Cardiovascular Risk in Diabetes BP trial (ACCORD BP) randomly assigned 4,733 participants with type 2 diabetes mellitus and HTN to a target SBP of either less than 120 mm Hg (the intensive group) or to less than 140 mm Hg (the standard group).[36] A variety of FDA-approved BP medications were used to reach BP goals. After an average follow-up of about 5 years, researchers found no significant differences between the intensive group and the standard group in rates of a combined endpoint including nonfatal heart attack, nonfatal stroke, or CV death. Lowering BP to below the standard level did, however, significantly cut the risk of stroke alone by about 40%. Patients in the intensive BP group had 36 strokes, compared to 62 strokes in the standard group. The researchers cautioned, however, that participants in the intensive BP group were more likely to have complications such as abnormally low BP or high levels of blood potassium. In addition, some laboratory measures of kidney function were worse in the intensive therapy group, but there was no difference in the rates of kidney failure (Fig. 5d.5).

Management of HTN and CKD

Antihypertensive treatment has been shown to reduce the rate of progression of glomerular disease in individuals with CKD.[37] The National Kidney Foundation's Kidney Disease Outcomes Quality Initiative (KDOQI) guidelines

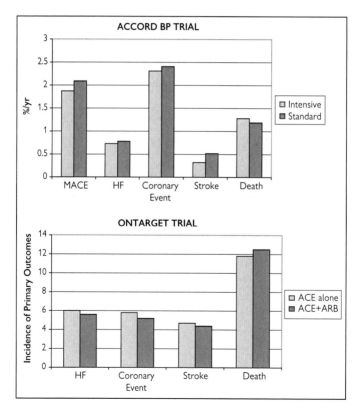

Figure 5d.5 Summary of findings from ACCORD BP and ONTARGET trials showing no benefit from intensive BP control or dual ACE inhibitor and ARB therapy.

recommend screening all patients with CKD for HTN, as they are considered the highest-risk group for CVD. Strict BP control is emphasized as the cornerstone of medical management in this group of individuals. These sets of patients should be held to a stricter BP goal of less than 130/80 mm Hg in the absence of proteinuria, or less than 125/75 mm Hg with proteinuria. Available evidence suggests that ACE inhibitors are more efficacious in slowing progression than can be explained by lowering of systemic BP alone[38,39] and that lowering BP within the normotensive range, which usually requires more than three agents, further reduces the rate of progression.[40] Most patients with CKD should receive an ACE inhibitor or an ARB in combination with a diuretic, and many will require a loop diuretic rather than a thiazide. Ambulatory BP monitoring and impedance cardiography measurement have recently been shown to augment therapeutic decision-making in the treatment of this select population with difficult-to-control HTN (Table 5d.1).[41,42]

KDOQI guidelines recommend that "individuals at increased risk of developing chronic kidney disease should undergo testing for markers of kidney damage," specifically for albuminuria. This is because a meta-analysis of individuals with CKD (eGFR <60 ml/min) and albuminuria found that positive predictors of outcome were lower SBP levels (110–129 mm Hg), lower albumin excretion (<1000mg/day), and the presence of ACE inhibitor therapy. These concepts of classification have been updated and put into an integrated risk map that is part of the KDIGO 2010 update of the classification system.[43] These updates indicate that anyone with an eGFR <45 ml/min coupled with more than 300 mg/day or more of albuminuria need aggressive risk factor management of blood pressure to levels <130/80 mm Hg, glucose (HbA1c <7%) and cholesterol per the SHARP trial to LDL <70 mg/dl to maximally reduce cardiovascular risk and CKD progression .[10,44,45]

Table 5d.1 Therapeutic Goals and Considerations for Compelling Indications

Area of concern	BP Target (mm Hg)	Lifestyle[†] modification	Specific Drug Indications
General CAD prevention	<140/90	Yes	Any effective antihypertensive drug or combination[‡]
High CAD risk*	<130/80	Yes	ACEI or ARB or CCB or thiazide or combination
Stable angina	<130/80	Yes	B-blocker and ACEI or ARB
UA/NSTEMI	<130/80	Yes	B-blocker and ACEI or ARB[§]
STEMI	<130/80	Yes	B-blocker and ACEI or ARB[§]
LVD	<130/80	Yes	ACEI or ARB and B-blocker and aldo antagonist and thiazide or loop diuretic and hydral/nitrate (blacks)

* diabetes, CKD, CAD or equivalent

[†] weight loss if appropriate, healthy diet, exercise, smoking cessation and alcohol moderation

[‡] evidence supports ACEI or ARB, CCB, or thiazide as first-line

[§] if anterior MI is present, if HTN persists, if LVD or HF is present, if diabetic

References

1. Vassalotti JA, Stevens LA, et al. Testing for chronic kidney disease: a position statement from the National Kidney Foundation. *Am J Kidney Dis* 2007;50(2):169–180.

2. Coresh J, Selvin E, et al. Prevalence of chronic kidney disease in the United States. *JAMA* 2007;298(17):2038–2047.

3. Klag MJ, Whelton PK, et al. Blood pressure and end-stage renal disease in men. *N Engl J Med* 1996;334(1):13–18.

4. Perneger TV, Whelton PK, et al. History of hypertension in patients treated for end-stage renal disease. *J Hypertens* 1997;15(4):451–456.

5. Perry HM Jr, Miller JP, et al. Early predictors of 15-year end-stage renal disease in hypertensive patients. *Hypertension* 1995;25(4 Pt 1):587–594.

6. Lubanski MS, McCullough PA. Kidney's role in hypertension. *Minerva Cardioangiol* 2009;57(6):743–759.

7. Sinclair AM, Isles CG, et al. Secondary hypertension in a blood pressure clinic. *Arch Intern Med* 1987;147(7):1289–1293.

8. Buckalew VM Jr, Berg RL, et al. Prevalence of hypertension in 1,795 subjects with chronic renal disease: the modification of diet in renal disease study baseline cohort. Modification of Diet in Renal Disease Study Group. *Am J Kidney Dis* 1996;28(6):811–821.

9. Hsu CY, McCulloch CE, et al. Elevated blood pressure and risk of end-stage renal disease in subjects without baseline kidney disease. *Arch Intern Med* 2005;165(8):923–928.

10. Jafar TH, Schmid CH, et al. Angiotensin-converting enzyme inhibitors and progression of nondiabetic renal disease. A meta-analysis of patient-level data. *Ann Intern Med* 2001;135(2):73–87.

11. Lackland DT, Egan BM, et al. Thirty-year survival for black and white hypertensive individuals in the Evans County Heart Study and the Hypertension Detection and Follow-up Program. *J Am Soc Hypertens* 2008;2(6):448–454.

12. Rosansky SJ, Hoover DR, et al. The association of blood pressure levels and change in renal function in hypertensive and nonhypertensive subjects. *Arch Intern Med* 1990;150(10):2073–2076.

13. Schaeffner ES, Kurth T, et al. Blood pressure measures and risk of chronic kidney disease in men. *Nephrol Dial Transplant* 2008;23(4):1246–1251.

14. Bakris GL, Williams M, et al. Preserving renal function in adults with hypertension and diabetes: a consensus approach. National Kidney Foundation Hypertension and Diabetes Executive Committees Working Group. *Am J Kidney Dis* 2000;36(3):646–661.

15. Young JH, Klag MJ, et al. Blood pressure and decline in kidney function: findings from the Systolic Hypertension in the Elderly Program (SHEP). *J Am Soc Nephrol* 2002;13(11):2776–2782.

16. Tracy RE. The heterogeneity of vascular findings in the kidneys of patients with benign essential hypertension. *Nephrol Dial Transplant* 1999;14(7):1634–1639.

17. Tracy RE, Lanjewar DN, et al. Renovasculopathies in elderly normotensives of Bombay, India. *Geriatr Nephrol Urol* 1997;7(2):101–109.

18. Johnson RJ, Gordon KL, et al. Renal injury and salt-sensitive hypertension after exposure to catecholamines. *Hypertension* 1999;34(1):151–159.

19. Franco M, Tapia E, et al. Renal cortical vasoconstriction contributes to development of salt-sensitive hypertension after angiotensin II exposure. *J Am Soc Nephrol* 2001;12(11):2263–2271.

20. Ballew JR, Fink GD. Role of endothelin ETB receptor activation in angiotensin II-induced hypertension: effects of salt intake. *Am J Physiol Heart Circ Physiol* 2001;281(5):H2218–2225.

21. Verhagen AM, Braam B, et al. Losartan-sensitive renal damage caused by chronic NOS inhibition does not involve increased renal angiotensin II concentrations. *Kidney Int* 1999;56(1):222–231.

22. Fujiwara N, Osanai T, et al. Study on the relationship between plasma nitrite and nitrate level and salt sensitivity in human hypertension: modulation of nitric oxide synthesis by salt intake. *Circulation* 2000;101(8):856–861.

23. Yu HT. Progression of chronic renal failure. *Arch Intern Med* 2003;163(12):1417–1429.

24. Martinez-Maldonado M. Role of hypertension in the progression of chronic renal disease. *Nephrol Dial Transplant* 2001;16(Suppl 1):63–66.

25. Maschio G, Oldrizzi L, et al. Hypertension and progression of renal disease. *J Nephrol* 2000;13(3):225–227.

26. Pisoni R, Remuzzi G. How much must blood pressure be reduced in order to obtain the remission of chronic renal disease? *J Nephrol* 2000;13(3):228–231.

27. Taal MW, Brenner BM. Renoprotective benefits of RAS inhibition: from ACEI to angiotensin II antagonists. *Kidney Int* 2000;57(5):1803–1817.

28. Manjunath G, Tighiouart H, et al. Level of kidney function as a risk factor for atherosclerotic cardiovascular outcomes in the community. *J Am Coll Cardiol* 2003;41(1):47–55.

29. McCullough PA, Khan M, et al. Serum cystatin C in the estimation of glomerular filtration on chronic angiotensin-converting enzyme inhibitor therapy: an illustrative case report. *J Clin Hypertens (Greenwich)* 2009;11(11):651–655.

30. Koren-Morag N, Goldbourt U, et al. Renal dysfunction and risk of ischemic stroke or TIA in patients with cardiovascular disease. *Neurology* 2006;67(2):224–228.

31. Wannamethee SG, Shaper SG, et al. Serum creatinine concentration and risk of cardiovascular disease: a possible marker for increased risk of stroke. *Stroke* 1997;28(3):557–563.

32. Lawes CM, Bennett DA, et al. Blood pressure and stroke: an overview of published reviews. *Stroke* 2004;35(4):1024.

33. Weiner DE, Tighiouart H, et al. Lowest systolic blood pressure is associated with stroke in stages 3 to 4 chronic kidney disease. *J Am Soc Nephrol* 2007;18(3):960–966.

34. McCullough PA. Why is chronic kidney disease the spoiler for cardiovascular outcomes? *J Am Coll Cardiol* 2003;41(5):725–728.

35. Yusuf S, Teo KK, et al. Telmisartan, ramipril, or both in patients at high risk for vascular events. *N Engl J Med* 2008;358(15):1547–1559.

36. Cushman WC, Evans GW, et al. Effects of intensive blood-pressure control in type 2 diabetes mellitus. *N Engl J Med* 2010;362(17):1575–1585.

37. Mogensen CE. Progression of nephropathy in long-term diabetics with proteinuria and effect of initial anti-hypertensive treatment. *Scand J Clin Lab Invest* 1976;36(4):383–388.

38. Maschio G, Alberti D, et al. Effect of the angiotensin-converting-enzyme inhibitor benazepril on the progression of chronic renal insufficiency. The Angiotensin-Converting-Enzyme Inhibition in Progressive Renal Insufficiency Study Group. *N Engl J Med* 1996;334(15):939–945.

39. Randomised placebo-controlled trial of effect of ramipril on decline in glomerular filtration rate and risk of terminal renal failure in proteinuric, non-diabetic nephropathy. The GISEN Group (Gruppo Italiano di Studi Epidemiologici in Nefrologia). *Lancet* 1997;349(9069):1857–1863.

40. Klahr S, Levey AS, et al. The effects of dietary protein restriction and blood-pressure control on the progression of chronic renal disease. Modification of Diet in Renal Disease Study Group. *N Engl J Med* 1994;330(13):877–884.

41. Ferrario CM, Flack JM, et al. Individualizing hypertension treatment with impedance cardiography: a meta-analysis of published trials. *Ther Adv Cardiovasc Dis* 2010;4(1):5–16.

42. Williams B, Lacy PS, et al. Differential impact of blood pressure-lowering drugs on central aortic pressure and clinical outcomes: principal results of the Conduit Artery Function Evaluation (CAFE) study. *Circulation* 2006;113(9):1213–1225.

43. Levey AS, de Jong PE, et al. The definition, classification, and prognosis of chronic kidney disease: a KDIGO Controversies Conference report. *Kidney Int* 2011;80:17–28.

44. Baigent C, Landray MJ, Reith C, et al. The effects of lowering LDL cholesterol with simvastatin plus ezetimibe in patients with chronic kidney disease (Study of Heart and Renal Protection): a randomised placebo-controlled trial. **Lancet** 2011;377(9784):2181–2192.

45. Jafar TH, Stark PC, et al. Progression of chronic kidney disease: the role of blood pressure control, proteinuria, and angiotensin-converting enzyme inhibition: a patient-level meta-analysis. *Ann Intern Med* 2003;139(4):244–252.

e. Cerebrovascular Disease/Cognitive Function

Fernando D. Testai, MD, PhD and
Philip B. Gorelick, MD, MPH

Vascular cognitive impairment (VCI) and Alzheimer's disease (AD) were traditionally believed to be two unrelated conditions. VCI was considered a consequence of cerebrovascular disease affecting strategic areas of the brain, whereas AD was deemed a progressive neurodegenerative condition caused by the accumulation of amyloid beta-peptide (senile plaques) and hyperphosphorylated microtubule-associated tau protein (neurofibrillary tangles). This paradigm, however, has been more recently challenged because VCI and AD neuropathologic changes may coexist and vascular risk factors may be important in the pathogenesis of both conditions. The introduction of modifiable vascular components in the genesis of VCI and AD has important potential practical implications for prevention and in addition shifts the pathophysiologic paradigm, particularly for those with early AD. In this section we will briefly review the relationship between these two types of dementia and their linkage to traditional vascular risk factors, including HTN, diabetes mellitus, and dyslipidemia.

HTN

The relationship between HTN and cognitive decline is not completely understood. Variations in study design, heterogeneous definition and assessment of cognitive impairment, and disparate interventions are just some of the variables that limit comparison among studies. Nonetheless, there is significant evidence supporting the role of HTN in the pathogenesis of cognitive impairment. Several epidemiologic studies illustrate this concept. In the Honolulu-Asia Aging Study, for example, the risk of poor cognitive function later in life increased by 9% for every 10-mm Hg increase in SBP in midlife, and the incidence of vascular dementia (VaD) and AD was approximately four times higher in untreated hypertensive individuals.[1,2] Midlife HTN was also a predictor of cognitive impairment is the Atherosclerosis Risk in Communities (ARIC) study, the Maine–Syracuse Longitudinal Study of Hypertension, and the National Heart, Lung, and Blood Institute Twin Study, among others.[3–5] Late-life HTN has also been linked to cognitive decline. In the Framingham heart study, chronic HTN was a predictor of attention and memory loss in middle-age and elderly (55 to 88 years) stroke-free individuals.[6] Similar results were observed in studies in Rotterdam, Göteborg, Uppsala, and Finland.[7–10]

The pathogenesis of cognitive impairment in hypertensive individuals is a matter of debate. The most simplistic mechanism suggests HTN may be linked to dementia by causing cerebrovascular damage to strategic areas of the brain involved in cognition. In the Rotterdam Scan Study silent thalamic infarcts were associated with memory loss and non-thalamic infarcts with psychomotor slowing.[11] The location of the affected area may be related to the type of dementia, with, for example, white matter lesions, nonlacunar infarcts, and left subcortical infarcts linked to VaD, and atrophy of the temporal sulci, dilated temporal horns and third ventricle, and right hemispheric infarcts on brain MRI associated with AD.[12,13] More striking is the suggestion that HTN and dementia share common pathogenic mechanisms, as pathologic (neurofibrillary tangles/ senile plaque density) and radiologic hallmarks (atrophy of the hippocampus and amygdala) of AD have been described in hypertensive individuals without dementia.[14,15]

The benefit of antihypertensive treatment in the prevention of cognitive impairment has yielded disparate results. The Hypertensive Old People in Edinburgh (HOPE) study showed that hypertensive treatment of older people with pre-existent cognitive impairment had no deleterious cognitive effects and may reverse cognitive impairment associated with pre-existent HTN. In the extended follow-up of Systolic Hypertension in Europe (Syst-Eur) study, BP treatment of non-demented hypertensive patients over 60 years of age reduced the risk of dementia by 55%.[16,17] In other studies involving cerebrovascular disease-free non-demented hypertensive patients, such as Systolic Hypertension in Elderly Prevention (SHEP), Study on Cognition and Prognosis in the Elderly (SCOPE), and Hypertension in the Very Elderly (HYVET) trials, the risk of cognitive decline was independent of the use of antihypertensive treatment.[18–20] Differential dropout, early termination, short follow-up, and inclusion of individuals with possible cognitive impairment at entry are some of the factors suggested to explain null results.[21] The findings may also be confounded by treatment intensity of HTN, as J- and U-shaped relationships between BP level and cognitive decline have been described.[22] It is hoped that the results of the ongoing multicenter study sponsored by the National Institutes of Health (NIH), Systolic Blood Pressure Intervention Trial (SPRINT), will clarify the potential benefit of aggressive BP treatment (SBP goal ≤120 mm Hg) in the reduction of age-related cognitive decline in individuals 55 years of age or older with baseline SBP at or above 130 mm Hg.

Diabetes Mellitus

Numerous epidemiologic studies have linked diabetes to cognitive impairment. In the Israeli Ischemic Heart Disease study, the rate of dementia three decades later in subjects with midlife diabetes was almost three times higher than in non-diabetic individuals.[23] Similarly, the Swedish Twin Registry showed that midlife diabetes was associated with an approximately twofold increased risk of dementia; these results were consistent for patients with VaD and AD subtypes.[24] Late-life diabetes has also been reported to be associated with dementia. In the Kungsholmen project, uncontrolled diabetes in subjects 75 years of age and older had a hazard ratio of almost three for VaD and AD compared to non-diabetic controls.[25] While the link between diabetes mellitus and VaD is generally accepted, its relationship with AD is not always consistent. The Framingham study, for example, did not show an association between diabetes mellitus and AD.[26] However, in the Columbia Aging Project the relative risk of AD and cognitive impairment without dementia in diabetic subjects was 1.6 compared to those without diabetes, and in the Uppsala Longitudinal Study of Adult Men, impaired insulin response in midlife was associated with increased risk of AD up to 35 years later.[27,28] Increased peripheral insulin levels have been associated with reduced AD-related brain atrophy, cognitive dysfunction, and dementia severity, suggesting that insulin may participate in the pathogenesis of AD.[29]

The expression of insulin receptors in areas of the brain responsible for cognition, such as the limbic system, suggests a role for insulin signaling in learning and long-term memory. Several pathogenic linkages support this hypothesis. First, insulin degrading enzyme plays a role in the degradation of amyloid beta-protein and amyloid precursor protein released by gamma-secretase activity, and acts synergistically with apoprotein E epsilon-4 by increasing the risk of late-onset AD,[30] and genetic alterations in or near the insulin degrading enzyme may be particularly associated with the occurrence of AD.[31] Second, more recently, the term *type 3 diabetes* has been coined; this is a particular type of neuroendocrine disorder found in AD patients that harbors elements of type 1 (decreased production of insulin) and type 2 (peripheral insulin resistance) diabetes.[32] It has been proposed that decreased insulin-mediated signaling dysregulates tau-protein production and leads ultimately to neuronal cell death and AD exacerbation. Amyloid beta-derived diffusible ligands have been described in AD and may participate in this process. These neurotoxic molecules contribute to lower insulin and to insulin resistance in AD brains as well as to other AD-related phenomenon such as oxidative damage and tau-protein hyperphosphorylation.[33] Third, the cholinergic hypothesis claims that AD is caused by inadequate production of acetylcholine. In this regard, insulin has been shown to stimulate the expression of choline acetyltransferase, a rate-limiting enzyme involved in the synthesis of acethylcholine.[34] Furthermore, it has been suggested that suboptimal insulin signaling is involved in lower production of acetylcholine in AD. Fourth, Advanced glycation end products (AGE) are heterogeneous non-ezymatically formed cross-linked sugar–protein complexes found in the central nervous system of diabetic patients. AGEs signal through specific membrane receptors called RAGE, and this interaction is modulated by a soluble decoy molecule called soluble-RAGE, which contains the RAGE ligand binding site but does not have a direct physiologic activity other than sequestering circulating AGE. The AGE/RAGE system is regarded as a putative risk factor for atherosclerosis, and its activation causes pro-inflammatory gene activation. The association between VaD and AGE is well established. In AD patients, AGE epitopes have been observed in areas of the brain involved in cognition, such as in the hippocampus and parahippocampal gyrus. AGE has also been identified in neurofibrillary tangles and senile plaques, suggesting its role in the pathogenesis of AD.[35]

These observations suggest that control of diabetes mellitus could possibly ameliorate or prevent cognitive decline. Among individuals with type 2 diabetes, a 1% increase in glycosylated hemoglobin level (HbA1c) was associated with a statistically significant decreased performance in neuropsychological testing (0.20-point lower Mini Mental Status Examination, 1.75-point lower Digit Symbol Substitution Test, and 0.11-point lower memory score).[36] In addition, in an autopsy study, the combination of insulin and other diabetes medications was associated with lower neuritic plaque density, a hallmark of AD neuropathology.[37]

The benefit of intensive glycemic control versus standard treatment (HbA1c ≤6 versus 7.0 to 7.9, respectively) in decreasing cognitive decline and structural brain changes in type 2 diabetic patients with traditional CV risk factors is being investigated in the NIH initiative Action to Control Cardiovascular Risk in Diabetes-Memory in Diabetes (ACCORD-MIND). This and other randomized placebo-controlled studies are necessary to determine the benefit of diabetes control in the prevention of cognitive decline.

Dyslipidemia

The role of lipid homeostasis in the development of cognitive decline is not completely understood. In a cohort of 1,111 non-demented subjects with mean age of 75 years, elevated low-density lipoprotein (LDL) cholesterol levels were associated with an approximately threefold increased relative risk of dementia with stroke compared to their counterparts with low LDL cholesterol levels.[38] In another study of 4,316 Medicare recipients at least 65 years of age, there was only a weak relationship between high-density lipoprotein (HDL) cholesterol, LDL cholesterol, and non-HDL cholesterol and the risk of VaD.[39] LDL cholesterol has also been linked to AD. In the Washington Heights/Inwood Columbia Aging Project, higher pre-diagnosis total cholesterol and LDL cholesterol and history of diabetes were associated with faster cognitive decline in patients with incident AD.[40] The results of studies that investigated the link between total cholesterol and risk for any type of dementia or AD, however, are conflicting. In the Honolulu-Asia aging study, for example, there was no correlation between total cholesterol and any type of dementia,[41] and in the Framingham study there was no correlation between total cholesterol and the risk of AD.[42]

On the other hand, some studies have found that elevated total cholesterol levels in the elderly (65 to 84 years of age) may have a protective effect against dementia.[43] These apparently contradictory results may be explained by the timing of cholesterol measurement in relation to age and onset of dementia. Midlife elevated cholesterol may be a risk for later cognitive impairment; however, this relationship may not hold in late life as cholesterol level decreases with age or as a result of cognitive decline.

Different mechanisms have been proposed to explain the possible link between cholesterol metabolism and cognitive dysfunction: (1) membrane cholesterol regulates amyloid precursor protein processing and may promote amyloidogenic processing via beta- and gamma-secretases instead of the non-amyloidogenic processing via alpha-secretase[44]; (2) there is increased production of oxysterols in AD brain, which may reflect oxidative stress and have a direct neurotoxic effect[45]; and (3) apolipoprotein E epsilon-4, which is associated with AD, binds aggregated amyloid beta-peptide, and both may impair NMDA-receptor mediated synaptic plasticity.[46]

The rate-limiting step in the synthesis of cholesterol is catalyzed by 3-hydroxy-3-methyglutaryl-CoA reductase. The use of inhibitors of this enzyme (statins) to prevent the development of dementia has led to mixed results. In a cross-sectional study, the prevalence of AD among those in the cohort taking statins was 60% to 73% ($p < 0.001$) lower than in the total population.[47] However, it is still unclear if these results are due to cholesterol-lowering properties of statins, or to one or more of the multiple pleiotropic functions of this drug class. The results obtained in the Boston Collaborative Drug Surveillance Program illustrate this concept. In this cohort, the use of statins in individuals at least 50 years of age lowered substantially the risk of dementia, independent of the presence or absence of untreated dyslipidemia or exposure to other lipid-lowering agents.[48]

While the results of these studies are promising, others have found no benefit associated with statins, and a recent Cochrane database review concluded that there is no solid evidence from randomized clinical trials supporting a role for this drug class in preventing cognitive decline.[49] Further investigations are necessary to understand the role of dyslipidemia in the pathogenesis of cognitive impairment and to determine the benefit of statin agents on preventing or reversing cognitive decline.

References

1. Launer LJ, Ross GW, Petrovitch H, Masaki K, Foley D, White LR, Havlik RJ. Midlife blood pressure and dementia: the Honolulu-Asia aging study. *Neurobiol Aging* 2000;21(1):49–55.

2. Launer LJ, Masaki K, Petrovitch H, Foley D, Havlik RJ. The association between midlife blood pressure levels and late-life cognitive function. The Honolulu-Asia Aging Study. *JAMA* 1995;274(23):1846–1851.

3. Knopman D, Boland LL, Mosley T, Howard G, Liao D, Szklo M, McGovern P, Folsom AR; Atherosclerosis Risk in Communities (ARIC) Study Investigators. Cardiovascular risk factors and cognitive decline in middle-aged adults. *Neurology* 2001;56(1):42–48.

4. Elias PK, Elias MF, Robbins MA, Budge MM. Blood pressure-related cognitive decline: does age make a difference? *Hypertension* 2004;44(5):631–636.

5. Swan GE, DeCarli C, Miller BL, Reed T, Wolf PA, Jack LM, Carmelli D. Association of midlife blood pressure to late-life cognitive decline and brain morphology. *Neurology* 1998;51(4):986–993.

6. Elias MF, Wolf PA, D'Agostino RB, Cobb J, White LR. Untreated blood pressure level is inversely related to cognitive functioning: the Framingham Study. *Am J Epidemiol* 1993;138(6):353–364.

7. Breteler MM, van Swieten JC, Bots ML, Grobbee DE, Claus JJ, van den Hout JH, van Harskamp F, Tanghe HL, de Jong PT, van Gijn J, et al. Cerebral white matter lesions, vascular risk factors, and cognitive function in a population-based study: the Rotterdam Study. *Neurology* 1994;44(7):1246–1252.

8. Skoog I, Lernfelt B, Landahl S, Palmertz B, Andreasson LA, Nilsson L, Persson G, Odén A, Svanborg A. 15-year longitudinal study of blood pressure and dementia. *Lancet* 1996;347:1141–1145.

9. Kilander L, Nyman H, Boberg M, Hansson L, Lithell H. Hypertension is related to cognitive impairment: a 20-year follow-up of 999 men. *Hypertension* 1998;31:780–786.

10. Kivipelto M, Helkala EL, Hänninen T, Laakso MP, Hallikainen M, Alhainen K, Soininen H, Tuomilehto J, Nissinen A. Midlife vascular risk factors and late-life mild cognitive impairment: A population-based study. *Neurology* 2001;56:1683–1689.

11. Vermeer SE, Prins ND, den Heijer T, Hofman A, Koudstaal PJ, Breteler MM. Silent brain infarcts and the risk of dementia and cognitive decline. *N Engl J Med* 2003;348(13):1215–1222.

12. den Heijer T, Launer LJ, Prins ND, van Dijk EJ, Vermeer SE, Hofman A, Koudstaal PJ, Breteler MM. Association between blood pressure, white matter lesions, and atrophy of the medial temporal lobe. *Neurology* 2005;64(2):263–267.

13. Charletta D, Gorelick PB, Dollear TJ, Freels S, Harris Y. CT and MRI findings among African-Americans with Alzheimer's disease, vascular dementia, and stroke without dementia. *Neurology* 1995;45(8):1456–1461.

14. Petrovitch H, White LR, Izmirilian G, Ross GW, Havlik RJ, Markesbery W, Nelson J, Davis DG, Hardman J, Foley DJ, Launer LJ. Midlife blood pressure and neuritic plaques, neurofibrillary tangles, and brain weight at death: the HAAS. Honolulu-Asia aging Study. *Neurobiol Aging* 2000;21:57–62.

15. den Heijer T, Launer LJ, Prins ND, van Dijk EJ, Vermeer SE, Hofman A, Koudstaal PJ, Breteler MM. Association between blood pressure, white matter lesions, and atrophy of the medial temporal lobe. *Neurology* 2005;64:263–267.

16. Starr JM, Whalley LJ, Deary IJ. The effects of antihypertensive treatment on cognitive function: results from the HOPE study. *J Am Geriatr Soc* 1996;44(4):411–415.

17. Forette F, Seux ML, Staessen JA, Thijs L, Babarskiene MR, Babeanu S, Bossini A, Fagard R, Gil-Extremera B, Laks T, Kobalava Z, Sarti C, Tuomilehto J, Vanhanen H, Webster J, Yodfat Y, Birkenhäger WH; Systolic Hypertension in Europe Investigators. The prevention of dementia with antihypertensive treatment: new evidence from the Systolic Hypertension in Europe (Syst-Eur) study. *Arch Intern Med* 2002;162(18):2046–2052.

18. Systolic Hypertension in the Elderly Program (SHEP) Cooperative Research Group. Prevention of stroke by antihypertensive drug treatment in older persons with isolated systolic hypertension. Final results of the SHEP. *JAMA* 1991;265:3255–3264.

19. Lithell H, Hansson L, Skoog I, Elmfeldt D, Hofman A, Olofsson B, Trenkwalder P, Zanchetti A; SCOPE Study Group. The Study on Cognition and Prognosis in the Elderly (SCOPE): principal results of a randomized double-blind intervention trial. *J Hypertens* 2003;21:875–886.

20. Peters R, Beckett N, Forette F, Tuomilehto J, Clarke R, Ritchie C, Waldman A, Walton I, Poulter R, Ma S, Comsa M, Burch L, Fletcher A, Bulpitt C; HYVET investigators. Incident dementia and blood pressure lowering in the Hypertension in the Very Elderly Trial cognitive function assessment (HYVET-COG): a double-blind, placebo controlled trial. *Lancet Neurol* 2008;7:683–689.

21. McGuinness B, Todd S, Passmore P, Bullock R. Blood pressure lowering in patients without prior cerebrovascular disease for prevention of cognitive impairment and dementia. *Cochrane Database Syst Rev* 2009 Oct 7;(4):CD004034.

22. Birns J, Kalra L. Cognitive function and hypertension. *J Hum Hypertens* 2009;23(2):86–96.

23. Schnaider Beeri M, Goldbourt U, Silverman JM, Noy S, Schmeidler J, Ravona-Springer R, Sverdlick A, Davidson M. Diabetes mellitus in midlife and the risk of dementia three decades later. *Neurology* 2004;63(10):1902–1907.

24. Xu W, Qiu C, Gatz M, Pedersen NL, Johansson B, Fratiglioni L. Mid- and late-life diabetes in relation to the risk of dementia: a population-based twin study. *Diabetes* 2009; 58(1):71–77.

25. Xu WL, von Strauss E, Qiu CX, Winblad B, Fratiglioni L. Uncontrolled diabetes increases the risk of Alzheimer's disease: a population-based cohort study. *Diabetologia* 2009;52(6):1031–1039.

26. Akomolafe A, Beiser A, Meigs JB, Au R, Green RC, Farrer LA, Wolf PA, Seshadri S. Diabetes mellitus and risk of developing Alzheimer disease: results from the Framingham Study. *Arch Neurol* 2006;63(11):1551–1555.

27. Luchsinger JA, Tang MX, Stern Y, Shea S, Mayeux R. Diabetes mellitus and risk of Alzheimer's disease and dementia with stroke in a multiethnic cohort. *Am J Epidemiol* 2001;154(7):635–641.

28. Rönnemaa E, Zethelius B, Sundelöf J, Sundström J, Degerman-Gunnarsson M, Berne C, Lannfelt L, Kilander L. Impaired insulin secretion increases the risk of Alzheimer disease. *Neurology* 2008;71(14):1065–1071.

29. Burns JM, Donnelly JE, Anderson HS, Mayo MS, Spencer-Gardner L, Thomas G, Cronk BB, Haddad Z, Klima D, Hansen D, Brooks WM. Peripheral insulin and brain structure in early Alzheimer disease. *Neurology* 2007;69(11):1094–1104.

30. Bian L, Yang JD, Guo TW, Sun Y, Duan SW, Chen WY, Pan YX, Feng GY, He L. Insulin-degrading enzyme and Alzheimer disease: a genetic association study in the Han Chinese. *Neurology* 2004;63(2):241–245.

31. Vepsäläinen S, Parkinson M, Helisalmi S, Mannermaa A, Soininen H, Tanzi RE, Bertram L, Hiltunen M. Insulin-degrading enzyme is genetically associated with Alzheimer's disease in the Finnish population. *J Med Genet* 2007;44(9):606–608.

32. Steen E, Terry BM, Rivera EJ, Cannon JL, Neely TR, Tavares R, Xu XJ, Wands JR, de la Monte SM. Impaired insulin and insulin-like growth factor expression and signaling mechanisms in Alzheimer's disease—is this type 3 diabetes? *J Alzheimers Dis* 2005;7(1):63–80.

33. De Felice FG, Wu D, Lambert MP, Fernandez SJ, Velasco PT, Lacor PN, Bigio EH, Jerecic J, Acton PJ, Shughrue PJ, Chen-Dodson E, Kinney GG, Klein WL. Alzheimer's disease-type neuronal tau hyperphosphorylation induced by A beta oligomers. *Neurobiol Aging* 2008;29(9):1334–1347.

34. Rivera EJ, Goldin A, Fulmer N, Tavares R, Wands JR, de la Monte SM. Insulin and insulin-like growth factor expression and function deteriorate with progression of Alzheimer's disease: link to brain reductions in acetylcholine. *J Alzheimers Dis* 2005;8(3):247–268.

35. Takeuchi M, Kikuchi S, Sasaki N, Suzuki T, Watai T, Iwaki M, Bucala R, Yamagishi S. Involvement of advanced glycation end-products (AGEs) in Alzheimer's disease. *Curr Alzheimer Res* 2004;1(1):39–46.

36. Cukierman-Yaffe T, Gerstein HC, Williamson JD, Lazar RM, Lovato L, Miller ME, Cok LH, Murray A, Sullivan MD, Marcovina SM, Launer LJ; Action to Control Cardiovascular Risk in Diabetes-Memory in Diabetes (ACCORD-MIND) Investigators. Relationship between baseline glycemic control and cognitive function in individuals with type 2 diabetes and other cardiovascular risk factors: the action to control cardiovascular risk in diabetes-memory in diabetes (ACCORD-MIND) trial. *Diabetes Care* 2009;32(2):221–226.

37. Beeri MS, Schmeidler J, Silverman JM, Gandy S, Wysocki M, Hannigan CM, Purohit DP, Lesser G, Grossman HT, Haroutunian V. Insulin in combination with other diabetes medication is associated with less Alzheimer neuropathology. *Neurology* 2008;71(10):750–757.

38. Moroney JT, Tang MX, Berglund L, Small S, Merchant C, Bell K, Stern Y, Mayeux R. Low-density lipoprotein cholesterol and the risk of dementia with stroke. *JAMA* 1999;282(3):254–260.

39. Reitz C, Tang MX, Luchsinger J, Mayeux R. Relation of plasma lipids to Alzheimer disease and vascular dementia. *Arch Neurol* 2004;61(5):705–714.

40. Helzner EP, Luchsinger JA, Scarmeas N, Cosentino S, Brickman AM, Glymour MM, Stern Y. Contribution of vascular risk factors to the progression in Alzheimer disease. *Arch Neurol* 2009;66(3):343–348.

41. Kalmijn S, Foley D, White L, Burchfiel CM, Curb JD, Petrovitch H, Ross GW, Havlik RJ, Launer LJ. Metabolic cardiovascular syndrome and risk of dementia in Japanese-American elderly men. The Honolulu-Asia aging study. *Arterioscler Thromb Vasc Biol* 2000;20(10):2255–2260.

42. Tan ZS, Seshadri S, Beiser A, Wilson PW, Kiel DP, Tocco M, D'Agostino RB, Wolf PA. Plasma total cholesterol level as a risk factor for Alzheimer disease: the Framingham Study. *Arch Intern Med.* 2003;163(9):1053–1057.

43. Solfrizzi V, Panza F, Colacicco AM, D'Introno A, Capurso C, Torres F, Grigoletto F, Maggi S, Del Parigi A, Reiman EM, Caselli RJ, Scafato E, Farchi G, Capurso A; Italian Longitudinal Study on Aging Working Group. Vascular risk factors, incidence of MCI, and rates of progression to dementia. *Neurology* 2004;63(10):1882–1891.

44. Wahrle S, Das P, Nyborg AC, McLendon C, Shoji M, Kawarabayashi T, Younkin LH, Younkin SG, Golde TE. Cholesterol-dependent gamma-secretase activity in buoyant cholesterol-rich membrane microdomains. *Neurobiol Dis* 2002;9(1):11–23.

45. Chang JY, Liu LZ. Neurotoxicity of cholesterol oxides on cultured cerebellar granule cells. *Neurochem Int* 1998;32:317–323.

46. Herz J, Chen Y. Reelin, lipoprotein receptors and synaptic plasticity. *Nat Rev Neurosci* 2006;7:850–859.

47. Wolozin B, Kellman W, Ruosseau P, Celesia GG, Siegel G. Decreased prevalence of Alzheimer disease associated with 3-hydroxy-3-methylglutaryl coenzyme A reductase inhibitors. *Arch Neurol* 2000;57(10):1439–1443.

48. Jick H, Zornberg GL, Jick SS, Seshadri S, Drachman DA. Statins and the risk of dementia. *Lancet* 2000;356(9242):1627–1631.

49. McGuinness B, Craig D, Bullock R, Passmore P. Statins for the prevention of dementia. *Cochrane Database Syst Rev* 2009 Apr 15;(2):CD003160.

Chapter 6

Special Populations

a. Hypertensive Urgencies and Emergencies

William J. Elliott, MD, PhD

A 57-year-old man visited an ophthalmologist because of 12 hours of blurred vision in his left eye. He originally denied other symptoms, but later admitted to having dull, poorly localized headaches, particularly in the mornings, for the past week or so. The only abnormalities on direct ophthalmoscopy were three flame hemorrhages (the largest of which was <1 disc diameter from the macula) and bilateral papilledema. He was referred to an internist for further evaluation. His initial office BP was 260/154 mm Hg, so he was directly admitted to the hospital. He had no pertinent past medical history, took no medications, and had last seen a physician 12 years earlier. Physical examination was unremarkable except for a BP of 256/152 mm Hg (with a pulse rate of 68 and regular) and the ophthalmic findings. Abnormal laboratory studies included BUN/creatinine of 48/1.9 mg/dL (eGFR = 39 mL/min/1.73 m^2) and voltage criteria for LV hypertrophy (with strain) on ECG. Urinalysis showed 4+ proteinuria and 3+ hematuria on dipstick and 4 to 10 red blood cells per high-power field on microscopic examination. He received an intravenous infusion of fenoldopam mesylate (beginning at 0.1 mcg/kg/min), which was titrated stepwise over 30 minutes to 0.6 mcg/kg/mg, resulting in a BP of ~200–210/125–130 mm Hg, as determined by an automated oscillometric syphgmomanometer. After the first hour, the dose was increased and the BP descended to ~180/110 mm Hg. After 8 hours at this level, the hematuria resolved (simultaneous with increases in his urinary flow rate and creatinine clearance). Captopril and immediate-release verapamil were administered orally, and the intravenous infusion was tapered over 2 hours and discontinued shortly thereafter. Urine collected during the first 24 hours of hospitalization contained levels of vanillylmandelic acid and metanephrines that were within the reference ranges; renal ultrasound showed bilateral 8-cm kidneys and no renovascular abnormalities. Repeat ophthalmologic examination showed complete resolution of the papilledema and improvement in all retinal hemorrhages 48 hours after admission. He was discharged on the third hospital day with a BP of 150–160/90–100 mm Hg on lisinopril, torsemide, and verapamil. At 15 office visits over the next 4 years, his BP was 124–129/76–79 mm Hg on doxazosin 4 mg/day, lisinopril 40 mg/day, torsemide 20 mg/day, and verapamil 360 mg/day, with no adverse effects. His ECG improved and his renal function stabilized at 1.6 to 1.8 mg/dL (eGFR 41 to 47 mL/min/1.73 m^2).

Although excellent outcomes data exist for the outpatient treatment of chronic HTN, very few comparative studies have demonstrated significant long-term prevention of CV and renal events after acute treatment of very high BPs.[1,2] Several strategies (e.g., rapid reduction of BP with sublingual nifedipine capsules, lowering BP into the "normal" range) acutely increase the risk of adverse outcomes (including CV events), but optimal treatment strategies have not been well defined.[3] Longstanding tradition has arbitrarily divided clinical scenarios with or without acute, ongoing, target organ damage into *hypertensive emergencies* or *hypertensive urgencies*, respectively.[4-6] The former are usually treated in intensive care units with a rapidly titratable, short-acting antihypertensive agent (e.g., sodium nitroprusside) and close monitoring of the patient for adverse effects, while the intrinsic autoregulatory capacity of the CV system is re-established. Hypertensive urgencies, however, are usually treated in the emergency or outpatient department with oral medications, with further evaluation and chronic treatment occurring 1 to 3 days later in an office setting. Whether acute lowering of BP in hypertensive urgencies should achieve a specific target, or even be instituted at all, remains unproven,[7] but it has been widely adopted in many urgent care settings.

The absolute BP level does not distinguish between emergencies and urgencies. Patients who were previously normotensive can develop a hypertensive emergency with a systolic BP that is only 30 to 50 mm Hg higher than their usual and customary level (e.g., 160/100 in a pre-eclamptic woman). Conversely, some chronically hypertensive patients remain asymptomatic and might qualify as only hypertensive urgencies, even with a blood pressure above 250/150 mm Hg. Seldom, if ever, does such a high BP require hospitalization if there is no acute target organ damage.

Common Types of Hypertensive Emergencies

The diagnosis of a hypertensive emergency is something of a judgment call because some physicians might disagree about the need to immediately treat the patient with severely elevated BP and evidence of acute, progressive target organ damage. Nonetheless, the most common scenarios include:

- Hypertensive encephalopathy (typically a diagnosis of exclusion)
- Acute LV failure and/or pulmonary edema
- Subarachnoid or intracerebral hemorrhage
- Acute aortic dissection (for which the target blood pressure is <120/70 mm Hg, within 20 minutes)
- Acute MI or acute coronary syndrome
- Adrenergic crisis (e.g., pheochromocytoma, phencyclidine or cocaine overdose)
- Glomerulonephritis or acute renal failure
- Epistaxis, gross hematuria, or threatened suture lines after vascular surgery
- Eclampsia

Epidemiology of Hypertensive Emergencies and Urgencies

Unlike the case summarized above, most affected patients have a history of stage 2 HTN that has not been adequately treated, typically due to non-adherence to prescribed medications. Drug and alcohol abuse (including tobacco) and low socioeconomic or minority status are other risk factors. Large claims databases suggest that the incidence in the United States is about 1 to 2 per million population/year. Hospitalization for a hypertensive crisis has been suggested as an (inverse) indicator of the quality of outpatient care in large healthcare plans. During the last millennium, renovascular HTN was often found in patients with Keith-Wagener-Barker grade III (hemorrhages/exudates) or IV (frank papilledema) retinopathy; a recent case series has confirmed a higher-than-expected prevalence of secondary HTN in patients with hypertensive urgencies or emergencies.[8]

Goal of Therapy

The most important pathophysiologic principle in this condition is that the patient's vascular beds have had their autoregulatory capacity reset, with the pressure–flow curve shifted up and to the right, compared to normal, during the days to weeks before the medical encounter. This has allowed the patient, over time, to constrict, and to continue to deliver an appropriate (if not quite normal) flow of blood and oxygen, despite the very high BPs. The major goal of treatment is to gradually reduce the BP for a sufficient period to allow these vascular beds to adjust to the new, lower pressure, without causing a precipitous decline in blood flow, which could lead to ischemia and/or infarction.

Most authorities recommend admission to an intensive care unit,[3,5,6] although a method to monitor BP (intra-arterial line vs. automated oscillometric device), an intravenous line to deliver the antihypertensive agent, and an attentive physician can begin the process in the emergency department (and, in fact, continue and complete it on a general medical floor, as was the case presented above).

No trials have been done to establish a BP target,[2] but most authorities recommend a decrease in mean arterial pressure by about 10% in the first hour, and no more than 25% during the first 2 hours. Most patients tolerate a BP of about 160–180/100 mm Hg well after the first 2 hours or so, but the antihypertensive medication dose should be individualized, and reduced if deterioration occurs when the BP is decreased too fast or too far. After the BP has been stabilized (usually for 6 to 24 hours), intravenous antihypertensive therapy can be withdrawn after oral treatment is administered.

Treatment Options

Many intravenous drugs have been studied for the treatment of hypertensive emergencies:[9] nitroprusside, labetalol, nitroglycerin, enalaprilat, nicardipine, esmolol, fenoldopam, and clevidipine.[10] Although probably the least expensive and most widely available, nitroprusside generates toxic cyanide and thiocyanate, is contraindicated in pregnancy and in patients with tobacco amblyopia or Leber's optic atrophy, and typically is used with aluminum foil to shield it from light; an intra-arterial line is required by nursing protocols. Fenoldopam, a selective dopamine-1 agonist, has beneficial acute effects on renal function. The effects of labetalol, nicardipine, and enalaprilat are difficult to reverse if the dose must be quickly reduced.

Most rapid-acting oral antihypertensive drugs can be used for hypertensive urgencies, but clonidine loading (0.2 mg acutely, 0.1 mg hourly thereafter) and nifedipine capsules (often administered sublingually or "bite-and-swallow") have been studied most intensively. Each has its drawbacks: the former often leads to drowsiness and a missed office visit the next day; during the last millennium, the U.S. FDA denied the latter an indication for acute lowering of BP in the setting of hypertensive urgencies.

Summary

The patient with very elevated BP should be evaluated for signs or symptoms of acute, ongoing target organ damage, which should allow discrimination between a hypertensive emergency (which should be treated in the hospital with a rapidly acting, easily titratable intravenous antihypertensive medication) or a hypertensive urgency (which may or may not need acute treatment). Depending on the type of hypertensive emergency, lowering of mean arterial pressure by 10% to 15% in the first hour, followed by another 10% to 15% over the next few hours, generally safely resets the autoregulatory capacity of most vascular beds, permitting withdrawal of the intravenous agent in favor of oral therapy, which the patient should thereafter take chronically. Evaluation for secondary causes of HTN is still widely recommended for patients with a hypertensive emergency, although the yield is probably lower than it was in the last millennium. Prognosis depends on baseline renal function and chronic adherence to antihypertensive drug therapy, and can be excellent.

References

1. Vicek M, Bur A, Woisetschläger C, Herkner H, Laggner AN, Hirschl MM. Association between hypertensive urgencies and subsequent cardiovascular events in patients with hypertension. *J Hypertens* 2008;26:657–662.

2. Cherney D, Straus S. Management of patients with hypertensive urgencies and emergencies: A systematic review of the literature. *J Gen Intern Med* 2002;17:937–945.

3. Agabiti-Rosei E, Salvetti M, Farsang C. European Society of Hypertension Scientific Newsletter: Treatment of hypertensive urgencies and emergencies. *J Hypertens* 2006;24:2482–2485 (also available in *Blood Press* 2006;15:255–256).

4. Rodriguez MA, Kumar SK, De Caro M. Hypertensive crisis. *Cardiol Rev* 2010;18:102–107.

5. Aggarwal M, Khan IA. Hypertensive crisis: Hypertensive emergencies and urgencies. *Cardiol Clin* 2006;24:135–146.

6. Vaughan C, Delanty N. Hypertensive emergencies. *Lancet* 2000;356:411–417.

7. Flanigan JS, Vitberg D. Hypertensive emergency and severe hypertension: What to treat, who to treat, and how to treat. *Med Clin North Am* 2006;90:439–451.

8. Börgel J, Springer S, Ghafoor J, et al. Unrecognized secondary causes of hypertension in patients with hypertensive urgency/emergency: Prevalence and co-prevalence. *Clin Res Cardiol* 2010;99:499–506.

9. Perez MI, Musini VM. Pharmacologic interventions for hypertensive emergencies: A Cochrane systematic review. *J Hum Hypertens* 2008;22:596–907 (also available as *Cochrane Database Syst Rev* 2008 (Jan):23(1):CD003653).

10. Deeks ED, Keating GM, Kearn SJ. Clevidipine: A review of its use in the management of acute hypertension. *Am J Cardiovasc Drugs* 2009;9:117–134.

b. Minorities

Samar A. Nasser, PhD, PAC, MPH, Phillip Levy, MD, MPH, Manmeet M. Singh, MD, and John M. Flack, MD, MPH

HTN is a common disease entity in both Western and global populations. While the prevalence in some racial/ethnic groups exceeds that of the white population, HTN rates are increasing in virtually all demographic subsegments of the United States and are excessive overall. HTN awareness, treatment, and control varies significantly across U.S. racial/ethnic groups. Lifestyle is a major determinant of disease burden and is likely the predominant factor contributing to racial/ethnic differences in the epidemiology of HTN.

HTN infrequently exists in isolation, and concomitant risk-enhancing conditions such as diabetes mellitus are often present in those with elevated BP. Among persons with diabetes, both glycemic and BP control are important risk factors for diabetic retinopathy, a major cause of vision loss/blindness. Moreover, BP control has been shown to reduce the progression of diabetic retinopathy and the need for retinal photocoagulation. Obesity, a pervasive condition that is disproportionately manifest in non-white racial/ethnic groups, not only increases the risk for diabetes and heart failure but is also a major contributor to pharmacologic treatment resistance. As noted in a recent report from the National Health and Nutrition Examination Survey (NHANES), obesity-related HTN has increased over the past two decades, particularly in men.

Epidemiology of HTN, Treatment, and Control Rates

Mexican-Americans

Overall, Mexican-Americans had the lowest level of HTN (25.5%), as compared to non-Hispanic blacks, who had the highest level of HTN (42.0%) versus non-Hispanic whites (28.8%). NHANES (1999–2004) data indicate that overall HTN awareness is greater among non-Hispanic whites (69.1%) and non-Hispanic blacks (71.0%) compared with the Mexican-American population (61.3%). During 2005–2008, the overall age-adjusted prevalence of HTN control among persons with HTN aged 18 years and up was 43.7%, while during NHANES 2007–2008 blood pressure was controlled in an estimated 50.1% of all patients with HTN.[1] Non-Hispanic blacks had a lower occurrence of controlled BP (41.2%) in comparison to non-Hispanic whites (46.5%); however, Mexican-Americans had the most despondent control rates overall (31.8%).[1] On the other hand, treatment and control rates did improve significantly between these two NHANES assessment periods. Much work remains to be done in regards to improving awareness and treatment success in the Mexican-American population.

American Indians

Until recently Native Americans had a relatively low prevalence of HTN. According to data from the Behavioral Risk Factor Surveillance System (BRFSS), American Indians now have one of the highest prevalences of HTN, placing second only behind African-Americans. According to the Inter-Tribal Heart Project, the prevalence of HTN among users of the Indian Health Service clinics was 31% among Chippewa and Menominee Indians over 25 years of age.[2] The Strong Heart Study (SHS), the largest epidemiologic study of American Indians ever undertaken, confirmed this high incidence of HTN, revealing a 27% to 56% prevalence of HTN in men and women between the ages of 45 and 75 years.[3]

To ascertain the prevalence of chronic disease risk factors in American Indian/Alaska Native (AI/AN) people, the Alaska Education and Research Towards Health (EARTH) Study was completed between 2004 and 2006.[4] The EARTH study revealed that among men, the most common risk factor overall was pre-HTN (49%). Notably, men had significantly higher age-adjusted odds of HTN and pre-HTN than their female counterparts. Given the impact of obesity-related HTN, the EARTH study also reported that the prevalence of overweight and obesity among AI/AN women was remarkably high (78%) compared with all other ethnicities from NHANES (66%). Similar to the Framingham Heart Study, the Strong Heart Study also found pre-HTN to increase the likelihood of CV events by 80% in comparison to healthy, normotensive individuals.[5] Nevertheless, HTN appears to be on the rise in the American Indian population. Significant challenges appear to remain in regards to increasing the frequency of treatment as well as the ultimate control of BP.

Asian/Pacific Islander Americans

Among Asian/Pacific Islander Americans (APIAs), HTN is widespread. According to the National Health Interview Survey (NHIS) 2004–2006, of those adults who were told they have HTN, Filipinos contributed 27%, while Japanese included 25%; however, both Chinese and Korean adults were lower, at 17%.[6] Overall, the prevalence of HTN in Asian-Americans was 16.1%,[7] which was almost half that of Caucasian Americans (28.5%), according to NHANES 2004.[8] Also, the Multi-Ethnic Study of Atherosclerosis (MESA) found that the age-adjusted prevalence of HTN in Asian-Americans (Chinese) was 39%, which was comparable to Caucasians (38%) and Hispanics (42%), but less than in African-Americans (60%).[9]

Another study based in San Francisco in 2000 revealed that 41% of Chinese hypertensives were taking antihypertensive medication, but only 14% of them had their BP controlled (<140/90 mm Hg).[10] In a follow-up study in 2001, 46% of these hypertensives were taking their BP medication, and an improved 26.9% had their BP controlled (<140/90 mm Hg). According to a recent study by Wong et al.,[11] approximately half of the participants admitted to non-adherence with hypertension care. Similarly, a study based in Maryland found that among hypertensive Korean-Americans (aged 60 to89 years), only 33.6% were taking antihypertensive medication and even fewer (7.5%) were under control. These studies also reflect the findings of the Study of Women's Health Across the Nation (SWAN), where the prevalence of treatment of Chinese-American and Japanese-American HTN patients was 34.4% and 48.4%, respectively. Of the hypertensive patients in the SWAN study, 25% of the Chinese-Americans and 38.7% of the Japanese-Americans had their BP controlled (<140/90 mm Hg).[12] BP control and treatment rates in the APIA population are significantly inadequate, and the data reflect the need for drastic improvement in treatment and control rates.

African-Americans

HTN in African-Americans has been extensively studied and reported on. There has been a long-held and pervasive view that HTN in African-Americans represents a distinct entity from HTN in other groups, especially U.S. whites. This perception has been driven by the higher incidence, prevalence, and target-organ injury (e.g., LV hypertrophy, chronic kidney disease [CKD]) rates observed in African-Americans than whites.

In a recent NHANES report spanning the 1988–1994 and 1999–2004 survey periods, non-Hispanic blacks were found to have higher awareness (71.0%) and treatment (54.8%) rates compared to non-Hispanic whites and Mexican-Americans. HTN awareness rates improved between the two survey periods from 71.0% to 75% ($p < 0.05$), treatment rates from 54.8% to 65.1% ($p < 0.001$), and control rates from 24.0% to 33.4% ($p < 0.001$). Control rates improved significantly in both women and men; however, the larger increase in BP control occurred in non-Hispanic black men (16.6% to 29.9%). In examining changes over NHANES 1988–2008, the prevalence of HTN was greater in blacks versus whites ($p < 0.001$) and Hispanics ($p < 0.001$), although there was no difference between white and Hispanic groups ($p = 0.12$).[1] HTN awareness, treatment, the proportion of patients with HTN treated and controlled, and the proportion with HTN controlled improved over time in white, black, and Hispanic groups according to NHANES 1988–1994 to 1999–2008.[1] Thus, despite significant improvements in HTN awareness, treatment, and control, all remain suboptimal, especially the latter two.

African-Americans do manifest abnormal BP diurnal variation more often, meaning they lack the normal 10% to 20% dip in nighttime BP from daytime levels. Plausibly, this increased 24-hour BP burden results in greater pressure-related target-organ injury. Alternatively, it may be that the attenuated nocturnal decline in BP is a manifestation of target-organ injury, which tends to occur with greater frequency among African-Americans than whites. Such disparate target-organ damage may be related to divergence in microvascular and macrovascular dysfunction attributable to both endothelial- and non–endothelial-dependent mechanisms. In particular, the large, central blood vessels manifest more stiffness and have anatomically thicker walls and reduced vasodilatory capacity in African-Americans. Consequently, central aortic pressure, the systemic afterload to which the heart and brain circulations are exposed, is higher in African-Americans than in whites.

Adverse pressure-related clinical outcomes, including heart failure, stroke, CKD/end-stage renal disease, and retinopathy (especially in persons with diabetes), occur with significantly greater frequency in African-Americans than whites. There is considerable evidence that successful BP treatment reduces the risk of these undesirable clinical outcomes. Data regarding prevention of progressive loss of kidney function and end-stage renal disease (ESRD) with aggressive BP control are especially strong for African-Americans with non-diabetic nephropathy and urine albumin:creatinine ratios above 0.22 (~300 mg/d of urinary albumin excretion).

Treatment

Good and effective HTN treatment does not appreciably differ between racial/ethnic groups. Nevertheless, the practitioner will be faced with different challenges as well as different levels of evidence in support of various treatments and treatment strategies across racial/ethnic groups. Most of the racial/ethnic-specific treatment recommendations have been developed for African-Americans and whites. The International Society on Hypertension in Blacks (ISHIB) recently published an updated consensus statement on HTN treatment in African-Americans.[13]

It is imperative that all patients be appropriately risk-stratified prior to treatment. In other words, patients should receive sufficient evaluation to accurately determine their goal BP and to identify other CVD risk factors (e.g., diabetes, dyslipidemia). Clinicians should encourage patients to actively participate in their own care by informing them of their target BP level and promoting use of self-monitoring (including BP measurement). Typically the focus on racial/ethnic-specific treatments has been on pharmacologic agents. Nevertheless, dietary preferences/habits will vary widely within racial/ethnic groups as well as between them. Given the importance of lifestyle and diet modification for BP control, individual food preferences should be determined, with an attempt to modify them gradually over time rather than mandating adherence to an idealized diet that may not be feasible to adhere to over even the short term.

When BP is more than 15 to 20 mm Hg systolic and/or more than 10 mm Hg diastolic above goal, combination drug therapy should be strongly considered. In complex drug regimens, diuretics are indispensable. When BP is not at goal despite the use of two non-diuretic drugs, the most effective option is to add a diuretic that is appropriate to the level of kidney function. Avoid therapeutic inertia but do not titrate drugs too rapidly: once every 4 weeks is fast enough in most situations.

References

1. Egan BM, Zhao Y, Axon R. US trends in prevalence, awareness, treatment, and control of hypertension, 1988–2008. *JAMA* 2010;303(20):2043–2050.

2. Welch VL, Casper ML, Rith-Nagarajan SJ. Correlates of hypertension among Chippewa and Menominee Indians, the Inter-Tribal Heart Project. *Ethn Dis* 2002;12(3):398.

3. Howard BV, Lee ET, Yeh JL. Hypertension in adult American Indians: the Strong Heart Study. *Hypertension* 1996;28:256.

4. Redwood DG, Lanier AP, Johnston JM, Asay ED, Slattery ML. Chronic disease risk factors among Alaska Native and American Indian people, Alaska, 2004–2006. *Prev Chronic Dis* 2010;7(4):A85.

5. Zhang Y, Lee ET, Devereux RB, Yeh J, Best LG, Fabsitz RR, et al. Prehypertension, diabetes, and cardiovascular disease risk in a population-based sample: the Strong Heart Study. *Hypertension* 2006;47(3):410–414.

6. Barnes PM, Adams PF, Powell-Griner E. Health characteristics of the Asian adult population: United States, 2004–2006. *Adv Data* 2008;394:1–22.

7. Rosamond W, Flegal K, Friday G, et al. Heart disease and stroke statistics—2007 update: a report from the American Heart Association Statistics Committee and Stroke Statistics Subcommittee. *Circulation* 2007;**115**:e69–e171.

8. Ong KL, Cheung BM, Man YB, et al. Prevalence, awareness, treatment, and control of hypertension among United States adults 1999–2004. *Hypertension* 2007;49:69–75.

9. Kramer H, Cong H, Post W, et al. Racial/ethnic differences in hypertension and hypertension treatment and control in the Multi-Ethnic Study of Atherosclerosis. *Am J Hypertension* 2004;17:963.

10. Lau DS, Lee G, Wong CC, et al. Characterization of systemic hypertension in the San Francisco Chinese community. *Am J Cardiol* 2005;96:570–573.

11. Wong CC, Mouanoutoua V, Chen MJ, Gray K, Tseng W. Adherence with hypertension care among Hmong Americans. *J Community Health Nurs* 2005;22(3):143–156.

12. Lloyd-Jones DM, Sutton-Tyrrell K, Patel AS, et al. Ethnic variation in hypertension among premenopausal and perimenopausal women: study of women's health across the nation. *Hypertension* 2005;46:689–695.

13. Flack JM, Sica DA, Bakris G, Brown AL, Ferdinand KC, Grimm RH Jr, Hall WD, Jones WE, Kountz DS, Lea JP, Nasser S, Nesbitt SD, Saunders E, Scisney-Matlock M, Jamerson KA; International Society on Hypertension in Blacks. Management of high blood pressure in Blacks: an update of the International Society on Hypertension in Blacks consensus statement. *Hypertension* 2010;56(5):780–800.

c. Hypertension in Pregnancy

Gerda G. Zeeman, MD, PhD, F. Gary Cunningham, MD, FACOG, and Marshall D. Lindheimer, MD, FACP, FRCOG (London ad eundem)

> A 31-year-old nullipara with four previous early miscarriages presents during gestational week 22 with a blood pressure of 164/110 mm Hg and 3+ protein-uria by dipstick. She has never had HTN and her BPs earlier in gestation were 125/75 mm Hg, with a negative dipstick test for protein. There is no family history of HTN, connective tissue disorders, or renal disease. Her laboratory testing reveals hemoglobin 12 g/dL, platelet count 200,000/microL, serum creat-inine 0.7 mg/dL, uric acid 5.1 mg/dL, and serum albumin 2.8 g/dL; a liver enzyme panel including lactic acid dehydrogenase was normal; and serological tests to identify anticardiolipin antibody syndrome were negative. Ultrasound showed a normally grown fetus, normal appearing placenta and amniotic fluid index. An intravenous infusion of magnesium sulfate is started and labetalol is administered parenterally, and BP decreases to the 140/90-mm Hg range. A timed urine col-lection demonstrates 4.2 g/day of protein. You are consulted for your opinion of the differential diagnosis and any other laboratory tests to obtain. Importantly, your input is requested for the crucial question of whether the pregnancy is per-mitted to continue, as well as suggestions on management.

Some form of HTN complicates 5% to 7% of all pregnancies, and it is a leading cause of maternal and fetal morbidity and mortality worldwide. The most common and serious cause of high BP in pregnancy is the pregnancy-specific preeclampsia syndrome. This disorder, a risk factor for recurrent hypertensive disorders in sub-sequent pregnancies, is also a risk marker for CV disease later in life. This section summarizes the clinical spectrum of HTN in pregnancy, focusing mainly on the multifaceted clinical presentation of women with the preeclampsia syndrome.

CV and Volume Changes in Normal Pregnancy

Understanding HTN in pregnancy requires knowledge of the physiologic changes in normal gestation. Profound alterations in CV function and volume homeosta-sis begin rapidly during the first trimester, continue but more slowly in the sec-ond trimester, and plateau usually during the last trimester. These changes include a substantial increase in cardiac output (30% to 50%) and intravascular volume.[1] Coincidentally, systemic vascular resistance decreases and vascular compliance increases, each markedly, so that despite increments in both cardiac output and intravascular volume, BP actually decreases, reaching a nadir at ~26 weeks. Other changes include renal hyperfiltration (~35%) and marked stimulation of the RAAS.

    The clinical relevance of these changes is considerable. For example, undiag-nosed chronic HTN may be masked by the physiologic early gestational decrease in BP. The normal increase in glomerular filtration, which is paralleled by increments in creatinine clearance, results in a lower plasma creatinine concentration, and levels considered normal for nonpregnant populations may be actually high in pregnant women, where a value of 0.9 mg/dL is already suspect.

Classification of HTN in Pregnancy

A number of schemas have been proposed by various national and international societies and organizations to classify the hypertensive disorders in pregnancy. Here we use the classification adapted by the High Blood Pressure Education Program Working Group (NHBPEP), published in 2000,[2] and re-endorsed by the American Society of HTN (ASH) in its 2010 position paper.[3] It is similar to that proposed by the American College of Obstetricians and Gynecologists (ACOG)[4] but differs from position papers of several other national society recommendations, summarized in a recent *Lancet* review.[5] The NHBPEP, ASH, and ACOG definitions used here appear to be those most encountered in the literature, and more important this classification schema appears to us to be one easily used in clinical circumstances. It is meant to include any form of HTN recognized during pregnancy; cases are placed into one of four categories.

Preeclampsia/Eclampsia

Preeclampsia, the disorder most often associated with severe maternal and perinatal morbidity and mortality, is defined as the *de novo* appearance of both HTN and proteinuria after midgestation, more frequently near term. HTN is defined as SBP 140 mm Hg or higher and/or DBP 90 mm Hg or higher, preferably confirmed by two readings taken 4 to 6 hours apart. Proteinuria is defined qualitatively as a dipstick reading at least 1+, or quantitatively as at least 300 mg/24 hours. Not yet officially incorporated into many guidelines, a urinary protein/creatinine ratio of at least 0.3 in a spot urine sample is now considered by many as equal to at least 300 mg/24 hours.[6]

In women without a history of HTN preeclampsia is more common in nulliparas. Of importance, preeclampsia is not only a hypertensive disease; rather, it is a multisystem disorder of which HTN is only one finding. The syndrome may be heralded by rapid weight gain and edema and a variety of symptoms, including headache, nausea, and abdominal pain. Laboratory evaluation may disclose evidence of microangiopathic hemolysis along with thrombocytopenia and schistocytes on the blood smear. Serum levels of hepatic transaminases may be increasing, while rising creatinine levels indicate renal functional loss.

Numerous schemas have been proposed categorizing preeclampsia as mild or severe, with one example shown in Table 6c.1. However, a major caveat to their application is that the clinical picture of seemingly mild disease can suddenly deteriorate, and thus designations such as mild and severe can be clinically misleading.

A deceptive complication of preeclampsia, pure or superimposed (see below), is labeled the HELLP syndrome, an acronym for Hemolysis Elevated Liver enzymes, Low Platelets. Starting with seemingly small changes, it can progress within 24 hours to a life-threatening syndrome characterized by worsening of thrombocytopenia and impressively increasing serum levels of LDH and serum transaminases.[7]

Table 6c.1 Preeclampsia: Judging Severity[#]

	Less Severe	More Severe
Presentation	≥ Gestational wk 34	< Gestational wk 35
Diastolic BP	<100 mm Hg	>110 mm Hg
Headache	Absent	Present
Visual disturbances	Absent	Present
Abdominal pain	Absent	Present
Oliguria	Absent	Present
$S_{Creatinine}$ (GFR)	Normal	Elevated (decreasing)
LDH, AST	Normal	Nephrotic range (>3 g/24h)[†]
Nonreassuring fetal testing[‡]	Absent	Present

"The American College of Obstetrics and Gynecology bulletins utilize the terms mild and severe for our preferred less and more severe, so as to underscore diligence for any form of preeclampsia.

Abbreviations: AST, aspartate aminotransferase; BP, blood pressure; GFR, glomerular filtration rate; LDH, lactic acid dehydrogenase.

[#]Presence of convulsions (eclampsia), congestive heart failure, or pulmonary edema are always very ominous signs.

[†]Degree of proteinuria alone may not indicate seriousness unless accompanied by other ominous sign or symptom.

[‡]Growth restriction and adverse signs during periodic fetal testing including electronic monitoring and Doppler ultrasound.

(Reprinted from Lindheimer JC, Taler SJ, Cunningham FG. Hypertension in pregnancy. ASH position paper. *J Am Soc Hypertens* 2010;4:68–78, with permission from Elsevier.)

Eclampsia is the convulsive phase of the preeclampsia syndrome, characterized by generalized tonic-clonic seizures. While convulsions are often preceded by premonitory signs such as headache and visual disturbances, apprehension, nausea/vomiting, excitability, and hyperreflexia, eclampsia may develop suddenly without much warning. Most cases manifest antepartum, intrapartum, or within the first 24 hours postpartum, but convulsions may develop up to a week or so in the puerperium. Rarely, eclampsia has been reported to develop weeks after delivery.[8]

Chronic HTN

Women with a history of HTN predating pregnancy or in whom high BP is detected in the first half of gestation fall into this category. Most have essential HTN, usually non-severe (defined here as SBP and/or DBP 160/105 mm Hg or less). Their pregnancies are usually uncomplicated, but not invariably, and ~25% of these women develop superimposed preeclampsia (see below). Of note, the "official" definition of HTN (140/90 mm Hg) is probably too high given the physiological vasodilation of pregnancy, and as noted, some women with undiagnosed disease are recorded as normotensive because of the physiologic decrement of BP in early pregnancy. Pregnant women with a BP of 120/80 mm Hg or higher in the first trimester thus deserve more careful scrutiny, as they may have mild chronic HTN that will cause complications later in the pregnancy. A minority of women in this category have secondary HTN due to intrinsic renal disease, endocrinopathies, connective tissue disease, and vascular disorders. In such women, complications are common and pregnancy outcomes worse. Pheochromocytoma is rare but may initially present in pregnancy, with disastrous outcomes when unsuspected. When diagnosed, these patients have been managed either surgically or with medical treatment and with successful outcomes.

Similarly, in rare cases of Cushing syndrome HTN often worsens, and the fetal outcome is poor. Ironically, primary aldosteronism may improve because of the massive amounts of progesterone synthesized by the placenta. This hormone blocks the action of aldosterone and may lower BP as well as diminish abnormal potassium excretion. Collagen-vascular disease is associated with an increased prevalence of hypertensive disorders, and lupus, scleroderma, and periarteritis nodosa are associated with serious and fatal complications. Renovascular HTN is uncommon, but angioplasty and stent placement have been successfully performed in pregnant women with renal artery stenosis. Further discussion of secondary HTN, beyond the scope of this chapter, can be found in reference 9.

Chronic HTN with Superimposed Preeclampsia

As many as a fourth of pregnant women with chronic HTN develop superimposed preeclampsia, a diagnosis that is difficult to make by clinical criteria alone. Many clinicians use criteria such as development of *de novo* proteinuria after midgestation, or acceleration of either HTN and/or proteinuria. This, however, may be misleading because glomerular membrane permeability to protein increases in late gestation, and thus all pregnant women experience small increments in protein excretion, albeit within the normal range. For example, in women with chronic HTN and some degree of glomerulosclerosis, in whom the tubular reabsorption is already maximal and urinary excretion near the upper limits of normal, the increase may be more substantial.[6] The diagnosis becomes more certain in the presence of other systemic manifestations of the preeclampsia syndrome, such as abnormal hematologic changes or evidence for hepatic or renal involvement. There is promise that measurement of circulating antiangiogenic proteins and other markers may improve our accuracy in diagnosing superimposed preeclampsia. A useful caveat, however, is that when in doubt, manage the patient as if she has superimposed preeclampsia, the potentially more malicious and unforgiving complication.

Gestational HTN

This category includes women whose HTN does not meet criteria for the first three. The diagnosis is arrived at after the fact and is basically one of exclusion. Gestational HTN describes new-onset HTN in the absence of proteinuria presenting after midgestation, often near term. The HTN is usually mild to moderate, but more severe rises are occasionally encountered. Classification of gestational HTN requires that BP normalizes postpartum. If so, some label the entity "transient HTN." Conversely, if high BP persists, the diagnosis is changed to "chronic HTN."

At least in retrospect, gestational HTN appears to harbor two major populations: preeclamptics yet to manifest proteinuria (and indeed some eventually do) and women destined to develop remote essential HTN. In either case gestational HTN, like preeclampsia, is a risk marker for developing chronic HTN later in life.

Pathogenic Mechanisms in Preeclampsia

There are still many theories centered about the causes of preeclampsia, though research these past two decades have led to a better understanding, at least, of what is now thought to be a number of the probable cause of several preeclampsia phenotypes. A more complete discussion, beyond the scope of this chapter, may be found elsewhere.[5,10–12] For what are probably some of the more common phenotypic expressions of the preeclampsia syndrome, there are plausible theories that are focused on the placenta and describe the disorder in two stages. In the first, labeled the placental stage, the initiating cause results in the placenta producing factors (e.g., specific proteins, placental "debris") that enter the maternal circulation. The second stage, the maternal stage, is overt disease that depends not only on the action of these circulating factors, but also on the health and phenotype of the mother, including diseases that may affect the vasculature (such as preexisting cardiorenal disease, metabolic or genetic factors, and obesity).

The placental stage is believed to be triggered by abnormal placentation characterized by a faulty and incomplete endotrophoblastic invasion of the spiral arteries. Instead of becoming normally dilated flaccid vessels, they instead remain narrowed with an intact muscularis, thus impeding blood flow and resulting in a more hypoxic placental environment. Promising work as of 2012 involved the role of abnormal placental proteins, the secretion of which is stimulated by hypoxemia; their action is to inhibit angiogenesis. Two of these antiangiogenic factors (soluble Fms-like tyrosine kinase-1, and soluble endoglin) have been shown to produce a preeclampsia-like disease in rodents, while in pregnant women their concentrations have been shown to increase weeks to months before overt disease.[13] In essence, placentas in pregnancies destined to become complicated by preeclampsia are thought to overproduce these proteins, which are then found in abnormal concentrations in the maternal circulation. Neutralizing their actions is now being investigated in animal models, and in some studies this has reversed the disease in rodents.

Even if the role of these antiangiogenic proteins in causing phenotypic preeclampsia is confirmed, the underlying cause for their placental overproduction remains obscure, and here other areas of investigation are ongoing. One important consideration is that there likely are a number of causes of the preeclampsia syndrome. Areas under investigation include prostaglandins, endogenous digoxin-like molecules, immunologic mechanisms, agonistic autoantibodies to the angiotensin 1 receptor, inflammation, oxidative stress, mitochondrial pathology, genes sensitive to low-oxygen environments, and cardiovascular maladaptations to the pregnant state. Although there are ongoing studies of putative causes from deficiencies in essential nutrients, minerals, and vitamins, there are a number of studies performed in impoverished countries in which replacement ("prevention") schemes have shown minimal or no success.

Pathophysiology of the Preeclampsia Syndrome

It is important to recall that HTN is but one clinical facet of the preeclampsia syndrome. Increased BP appears to be stimulated by markedly increased systemic vascular resistance that results in marked vasoconstriction as both cardiac output and arterial compliance are reduced. This is in response to decreased intravascular volume from capillary endothelial damage with leakage into the extracellular space and extravasation of albumin causing lowered plasma oncotic pressure. This "leaky endothelium" leads to generalized edema. In most women, however, except in those with very severe disease and, especially eclampsia, intravascular volume remains above that in the nonpregnant state. The reduced vascular compliance could conceivably play some role in the pressure rise.

GFR decreases in preeclampsia, but as it rises markedly in normal gestation, creatinine levels often remain at or below nonpregnant levels. Occasionally acute renal failure and, rarely, acute cortical necrosis have been described. The decreased GFR has been ascribed to decrements in renal blood flow and to glomerular pathology. A characteristic swelling of the glomerular endothelial cell (termed endotheliosis) and decreases in available surface area for filtration (a decreased ultrafiltration coefficient [K_f]) have been implicated in the decrease in GFR.

Proteinuria, a diagnostic hallmark of preeclampsia, is ascribed to abnormal podocyte function. Of interest are animal model studies where glomerular endotheliosis and increased protein excretion can be produced by excess sFlt-tyrosine kinase, the soluble receptor to vascular endothelial growth factor (VEGF), and both the proteinuria and the glomerular endotheliosis can be reversed by administrating VEGF-125. Such observations further implicate antiangiogenic proteins to preeclampsia phenotypes.

Eclampsia with generalized seizure activity is the most recognizable cerebral manifestation of the preeclampsia syndrome. Commonly encountered symptoms include headache and scotomata. With the advent of sophisticated neuroimaging techniques, the cerebrovascular pathophysiology of the preeclampsia syndrome has been better elucidated when compared with previous neuroanatomic findings at autopsy. Imaging studies of patients who develop eclamptic convulsions reveal mostly transient changes compatible with localized edema, and often a pattern similar to that observed with the posterior reversible encephalopathy syndrome. Cerebral blood flow measurements done with MR imaging indicate hyperperfusion, which, when combined with the capillary endothelial leak described above, results in extravasation of fluid through the pericytes, and the resulting pericellular edema and capillary thromboses stimulate convulsions. Animal models have substantiated these findings and further show that normal autoregulation is not perceivably altered during pregnancy. Clinically this is a picture akin to hypertensive encephalopathy, except that preeclamptic women most often develop convulsions with BP far below those of typical patients with hypertensive encephalopathy. And here again, antiangiogenic proteins have been implicated in the cerebral pathology of animal models of preeclampsia.

Regarding the liver (see HELLP syndrome described above), organ changes range microscopically from a characteristic periportal lesion to macroscopic petechiae, as well as serious and potentially fatal subcapsular hematomas. Although immunofluorescence studies have shown widespread periportal fibrinogen/fibrin deposition, the preeclampsia syndrome is seldom accompanied by clinical evidence of consumptive coagulopathy and hypofibrinogenemia. Finally, there may also be substantial intracellular fatty changes, but these do not rise to the level seen with acute fatty liver of pregnancy.

Coagulation changes have been described in preeclampsia, but these generally are not clinically worrisome. For example, there is subtle and usually subclinical activation of coagulation; platelet stimulation and exhaustion with increased turnover and dysfunction; as well as other evidence for changes in the coagulation cascade. One concern is severe thrombocytopenia, usually seen in women with the HELLP syndrome described above, and platelet transfusions may be necessary if cesarean delivery or other operative procedures are planned.

Prediction and Prevention of Preeclampsia

Many trials evaluating tests to predict preeclampsia, or to distinguish it from more benign hypertensive conditions, have been reported, but no single test appeared clinically useful.[14] As of 2012, investigators have been focusing on combinations of tests, often including one or more antiangiogenic protein measurements. A few show promising results, with likelihood ratios acceptable for clinical use.

Countless interventions have been proposed to prevent preeclampsia, most but not all predicated on theories that a drug, mineral, vitamin, etc., will inhibit or reverse a presumed causal mechanism.[15] As of 2012, only two, low-dose aspirin treatment and dietary calcium supplementation, appear to be somewhat protective, but the numbers-needed-to-treat to prevent adverse outcomes are large.

Management of Hypertensive Disease in Pregnancy

Suspicion of preeclampsia is sufficient reason to recommend hospitalization, as seemingly mild disease may accelerate rapidly. Delivery remains the only known cure. Near term, induction of labor is preferred, but for preterm disease attempts to temporize may be justified if appropriate precautions are taken. However, delivery is indicated at any gestational age if severe HTN remains uncontrolled or if ominous findings appear, such as worsening liver abnormalities, decreasing renal function, signs of impending eclampsia, or development of nonreassuring fetal status as determined by a number of obstetric criteria. Because of this eventuality, severe preeclampsia remote from term should prompt hospitalization with close monitoring in specialized obstetric care centers.

Management of HTN

Decisions to treat HTN during pregnancy center on whether it is new-onset versus chronic HTN, its degree of severity, the gestational age, and importantly whether there is preeclampsia. Thus, there are unresolved issues regarding management of the hypertensive disorders of pregnancy. In addition, because uterine perfusion, and thus fetal perfusion, is flow-dependent and thus BP-related, there is concern as to how aggressively BP should be lowered. For example, there are likely significant differences in treatment of severe acutely elevated BP in contrast to chronic elevations encountered in managing women with chronic HTN. These exigencies have led to differing opinions on when to commence drug management and the levels of BP control to be attained.

Sudden Escalating HTN

There are two aims of lowering elevated BPs, especially if they are of recent onset and are increasing. With preeclampsia, this will lessen the likelihood of eclamptic seizures and cerebral edema. With chronic HTN, it protects against hemorrhagic strokes. Empirically, the NHBPEP[2] and ASH[3] documents recommend that a DBP of 105 mm Hg or above be treated. Although long suspected, only recently is there evidence that SBP of 160 mm Hg or more is associated with increased cerebral accidents; thus, such levels should be lowered, too.[16] Also, treatment is indicated at any level of symptomatic HTN (e.g., signs of cardiac decompensation, upper abdominal pain, and cerebral symptoms including severe headache, altered mental status, nausea/vomiting, and hyperreflexia). It is important to prevent precipitous BP decrements, or too low an endpoint, as either, and especially both in combination, may lead to fetal jeopardy, which might prompt emergency cesarean delivery in an unstable woman. Maintaining levels near 140–150/90–100 mm Hg in asymptomatic women seems ideal. Finally, as of 2012, the parenteral drugs most used to treat acute escalating HTN in pregnant women are hydralazine and labetalol (Table 6C2). Escalating HTN also requires eclampsia prophylaxis with magnesium sulfate ($MgSO_4$).[17]

Table 6c.2 Drugs for Urgent Control of Severe HTN in Pregnancy

Drug (Food and Drug Administration risk)*	Dose and Rate	Concerns or Comments#
Labetalol (C)	20 mg IV, then 20–80 mg every 20–30 min, up to a maximum of 300 mg; or constant infusion of 1–2 mg/min	Experience in pregnancy less than with hydralazine probably less risk for tachycardia and arrhythmia than with other vasodilators.
Hydralazine (C)	5 mg, IV or IM, then 5–10 mg every 20–40 min; or constant infusion of 0.5–10 mg/h	Drug of choice according to NHBEP working group; long experience of safety and efficacy.
Nifedipine (C)	Tablets recommended only; 10–30 mg orally, repeat in 45 min if needed	Possible interference with labor.
Relatively contraindicated nitroprusside (C)‡	Constant infusion of 0.5–10 µg/kg/min	Possible cyanide toxicity; agent of last resort.

*Indicated for acute increase of diastolic blood pressure ≥ 105 mm Hg; goal is a gradual reduction to 90/100 mm Hg.

C indicates that either studies in animals have revealed adverse effects on the fetus (teratogenic, embryocidal, or other), that there are no controlled studies in women, or studies in women and animals are not available. Drugs should be given only if the potential benefits justify the potential risk to the fetus.

Abbreviations: IM, intramuscularly; IV, intravenously; NHBEP, National High Blood Pressure Education Program.

*US Food and Drug Administration classification.

#Adverse effects for all agents, except as noted, may include headache, flushing, nausea, and tachycardia (primarily caused by precipitous hypotension and reflex sympathetic activation).

‡We would classify as category D; there is positive evidence of human fetal risk, but the benefits of use in pregnant women may be acceptable despite the risk (e.g., if the drug is needed in a life-threatening situation or for a serious disease for which safer drugs cannot be used or are ineffective)."

(Reprinted from Lindheimer JC, Taler SJ, Cunningham FG. Hypertension in pregnancy. ASH position paper. *J Am Soc Hypertens* 2010;4:68–78, with permission from Elsevier.)

Though there is universal agreement in the United States that MgSO$_4$ therapy should be commenced in situations like those discussed above, as well as in those with eclampsia, there is lack of unanimity as to when and whom to treat prophylactically. Intravenous MgSO$_4$ has some serious risks, and some contend they outweigh benefits in women with "mild" manifestations of the disease, reserving its use for situations deemed "severe." Given the capricious and explosive nature of preeclampsia, we consider administering MgSO$_4$ therapy in all patients suspected of having preeclampsia, but recommend its use in all of those with symptoms of severe preeclampsia. We further recommend its use for severe gestational HTN even when proteinuria appears absent. Note, however, there is controversy in that some withhold magnesium therapy when preeclampsia is considered mild, believing that the risks of the therapy outweigh prevention. However, recall that preeclampsia is an explosive disorder, making terms like "mild" misleading.

Chronic HTN

There are no consensus opinions concerning whether to treat women with HTN predating pregnancy, to continue treatment already being administered, or what BP levels are dangerous and unequivocally mandate treatment. That said, there is universal agreement that BPs considered in the severe range should be treated, and the debate focuses on women with mild to moderate rises in BP (Table 6C3). The reluctance to treat all degrees of chronic HTN with antihypertensive drugs relates to concerns for fetal safety as well as uncontested improved outcomes with versus without treatment.

Of note, all forms of chronic HTN are associated with increased incidences of earlier and severe superimposed preeclampsia as well as placental abruption, renal failure, cardiac decompensation, and cerebral hemorrhage. Adverse perinatal outcomes include stillbirth, growth restriction, and preterm delivery. Most of these adverse outcomes relate to the ~25% who develop superimposed preeclampsia. Unfortunately, systematic reviews of randomized trials of antihypertensive therapy in pregnant women with mild to moderate elevations of BP almost unanimously confirm that antihypertensive treatment with meaningful BP reduction does not seem to prevent superimposed preeclampsia.[9] Because of this, guidelines of both NHBPEP[2] and ACOG[4] consider treatment for mild or moderate HTN during pregnancy to be acceptable, but recommend beginning such treatment for women whose DBPs reach 100 mm Hg or higher. They go on to recommend, however, that women with evidence of end-organ damage (e.g., cardiac hypertrophy, renal dysfunction, chronic retinal changes) should be treated as aggressively as in the nonpregnant state. Also, as is the case with sudden escalation of HTN, treatment of severe systolic HTN (160 mm Hg or higher) is recommended to prevent cerebrovascular accidents.

Clinicians considering prescribing antihypertensive drugs should also be aware that many, if not most, of the reported randomized trials have limitations, and the area needs considerably more research. Still, Tables 6c.2 and 6c.3 summarize the status of several antihypertensive drug regimens in use during gestation, listing their pregnancy risk categories as defined by the U.S. FDA. The central adrenergic inhibitor methyldopa is listed as preferred, reflecting its more than 20 years of postmarket surveillance, several controlled trials, and the longest follow-up (7.5 years) in neonates. Another drug class commonly used is the combined alpha–beta-blocking agent, labetalol. Importantly, both ACE inhibitors and

Table 6c.3 Drugs for Chronic HTN in Pregnancy

Drug (Food and Drug Administration risk)*	Dose and Rate	Concerns or Comments
Methyldopa (B)	0.5–3.0 g/d in 2 divided doses	Drug of choice according to NHBEP working group; safety after first trimester well documented, including 7-year follow-up evaluation of offspring.
Labetalol (C)†	200–1200 mg/d in 2–3 divided doses	Gaining in popularity as concerns relating to growth restriction and neonatal bradycardia do not seem to have materialized.
Nifedipine (C)	30–120 mg/d of a slow-release preparation	May inhibit labor and have synergistic interaction with magnesium sulfate; small experience with other calcium-entry blockers.
Hydralazine (C)	50–300 mg/d in 2–4 divided doses	Few controlled trials, long experience with few adverse events documented, useful only in combination with sympatholytic agent; may cause neonatal thrombocytopenia.
β-receptor blockers (C)	Depends on specific agent	May cause fetal bradycardia and decrease uteroplacental blood flow, this effect may be less for agents with partial agonist activity; may impair fetal response to hypoxic stress; risk for growth retardation when started in first or second trimester (atenolol).
Hydrochlorothiazide (C)	25 mg/d	Majority of controlled studies in normotensive pregnant women rather than hypertensive patients, can cause volume depletion and electrolyte disorders; may be useful in combination with methyldopa and vasodilator to mitigate compensatory fluid retention.
Contraindicated ACE inhibitors and ATI-receptor antagonists (D)‡		Use associated with major anomalies plus fetopathy, oligohydramnios, growth restriction, and neonatal anuric renal failure, which may be fatal.

ACE, angiotensin-converting enzyme; NHBEP, National High Blood Pressure Education Program.

Note: No antihypertensive drug has been proven safe for use during the first trimester. Drug therapy is indicated for uncomplicated chronic hypertension when diastolic blood pressure is ≥ 100 mm Hg (Korotkoff V). Treatment at lower levels may be indicated for patients with diabetes mellitus, renal disease, or target organ damage.

* U.S. Food and Drug Administration classification

† We omit some agents (e.g., clonidine, α-blockers) because of limited data on use for chronic hypertension in pregnancy.

‡ We would classify in category X during second and third trimesters.

(Reprinted from Lindheimer JC, Taler SJ, Cunningham FG. Hypertension in pregnancy. ASH position paper. J Am Soc Hypertens 2010;4:68–78, with permission from Elsevier.)

ARBs should be avoided because they have been shown to be teratogenic for the embryo if exposed during the first 10 weeks of pregnancy, and they also cause fetal developmental abnormalities when given after the first trimester and even late in pregnancy. While listed in FDA Category D, most consider them contraindicated. Information on use of antihypertensive drugs during lactation remains limited. Drugs with high protein binding are preferred, such as labetalol. ACE inhibitors can be used as well. Diuretics may decrease breast milk production.

Obstetric Management Considerations

Methods to evaluate and monitor fetal well-being, delivery, and the use of analgesia and anesthesia for labor and delivery are beyond the scope of this chapter. The interested reader is referred to standard obstetric texts.[11,12]

Remote Prognosis

Results of several large epidemiologic studies have consistently shown that preeclampsia is a risk marker for developing CV, cerebrovascular, and metabolic disease later in life.[18] The risk is even greater for those who have early-onset preeclampsia (prior to 34 weeks) as well as women who have recurrent preeclampsia in more than one, but not necessarily consecutive, pregnancies. A reasonable interpretation is that preeclampsia is a risk marker of women predestined to have future CV or metabolic disease. In this regard, it is much like gestational diabetes predicting a high likelihood of overt diabetes developing years later. Such women, therefore, should have frequent health checkups and should be advised that lifestyle and dietary changes may minimize such problems in the future.

Case Study

The patient at the beginning of the chapter is drawn from a composite that exemplifies a relatively common consultation to many physicians who focus on the management of hypertensive patients, including requested advice from colleagues that obstetricians encounter.

The woman presented at 22 weeks' gestation, which is usually too early to temporize successfully if this is preeclampsia. The consultant should attempt to exclude other diseases in the differential diagnosis, focusing on exacerbations of multisystem disorders. In this particular case, the history of four consecutive early pregnancy losses may be associated with the lupus anticoagulant, with or without systemic lupus erythematosus. Other renal glomerular disorders, as well as other forms of secondary HTN, would be another consideration. It is hoped that measurement of angiogenic factors (which in 2011 was en route to becoming commercially available) will help considerably in the differential diagnosis.

In this case no evidence of other causes of HTN emerged, and though her BP was initially controlled, it rose again coincident with other multisystem signs of severe preeclampsia, and the gestation was terminated 6 days later. Within 24 hours her BP begin to decrease, she had an impressive diuresis, with a 10-kg weight loss by 3 days, and she was normotensive when seen for postpartum follow-up at 2 weeks. She is counseled about an increased likelihood of early recurrent preeclampsia in subsequent pregnancies as well as her increased risk for manifestation of lupus or another collagen-vascular disease.

References

1. Hibbard JU, Shroff SG, Lindheimer MD. Cardiovascular alterations in normal and abnormal pregnancy. In Lindheimer MD, Roberts JM, Cunningham FG, eds. *Chesley's Hypertensive Disorders in Pregnancy*, 3rd ed. San Diego: Elsevier Inc., 2009.

2. Report of the National High Blood Pressure Education Program Working Group on High Blood Pressure in Pregnancy. *Am J Obstet Gynecol* 2000;40:133–138.

3. Lindheimer JC, Taler SJ, Cunningham FG. Hypertension in pregnancy. ASH position paper. *J Am Soc Hypertens* 2010;4:68–78.

4. Diagnosis and management of preeclampsia and eclampsia. Number 33, January 2002. *Obstet Gynecol* 2002;99:159–167.

5. Steegers EAP, von Dadelszen, Duvekot JJ, Pijnenborg R. Pre-eclampsia. *Lancet* 2010;376(9741):631–644.

6. Lindheimer MD, Kanter D. Interpreting abnormal proteinuria in pregnancy. *Obstet Gynecol* 2010;115:365–375.

7. Sibai BM. Diagnosis, controversies, and management of the syndrome of hemolysis, elevated liver enzymes, and low platelet count. *Obstet Gynecol* 2004;103:981–991.

8. Hirshfeld-Cytron J, Lam C, Karumanchi SA, Lindheimer M. Late postpartum eclampsia: examples and review. *Obstet Gynecol Surv* 2006;61:471–480.

9. August P, Lindheimer MD. Chronic hypertension in pregnancy. In Lindheimer MD, Roberts JM, Cunningham FG, eds. *Chesley's Hypertensive Disorders in Pregnancy*, 3rd ed. San Diego: Elsevier Inc., 2009.

10. Hladunewich M, Karumanchi SA, Lafayette R. Pathophysiology of the clinical manifestations of preeclampsia. *Clin J Am Soc Nephrol* 2007;2:543–549.

11. Lindheimer MD, Roberts JM, Cunningham FG, eds. *Chesley's Hypertensive Disorders in Pregnancy*, 3rd ed. San Diego: Elsevier Inc., 2009.

12. Cunningham FG, Leveno KL, Bloom SL, Hauth JC, Rouse DJ, Spong CY. *Williams Obstetrics*, 23rd ed. McGraw-Hill, 2010.

13. Maynard SE, Karumanchi SA. Angiogenic factors and preeclampsia, *Semin Nephrol* 2011;31:33–46.

14. Conde-Agudelo A, Romero R, Lindheimer MD. Tests to predict preeclampsia. In Lindheimer MD, Roberts JM, Cunningham FG, eds. *Chesley's Hypertensive Disorders in Pregnancy*, 3rd ed. San Diego: Elsevier Inc., 2009.

15. Sibai BM, Cunningham FG. Prevention of preeclampsia and eclampsia. In Lindheimer MD, Roberts JM, Cunningham FG, eds. *Chesley's Hypertensive Disorders in Pregnancy*, 3rd ed. San Diego: Elsevier Inc., 2009.

16. Martin JN Jr., Thigpen BD, Moore RC, et al. Stroke and severe preeclampsia and eclampsia: a paradigm shift focusing on systolic blood pressure. *Obstet Gynecol* 2005;105:246–254.

17. World Health Organization. WHO recommendations for prevention and treatment of pre-eclampsia and eclampsia. WHO, Geneva, 2011. available at: www.who.int/reproductivehealth/publications/maternal_perinatal_health/9789241548335/en/index.html

18. Harskamp RE, Zeeman GG. Preeclampsia: at risk for remote cardiovascular disease. *Am J Med Sci* 2007;334:291–295.

d. Hypertension in Children and Adolescents

Bonita Falkner, MD

HTN may occur at any phase of childhood, from the newborn period through adolescence. Compared to HTN in adults, childhood HTN is defined differently and occurs less frequently. HTN in very young children, especially young children with marked BP elevations, is often secondary to an underlying disorder. In older children and adolescents, primary, or essential, HTN is more frequently the basis for the elevated BP. The prevalence of HTN in healthy asymptomatic children from age 3 to 18 years, based on recent data, is approximately 3.5%; the prevalence of prehypertension is also approximately 3.5%.[1,2] These rates are somewhat lower in younger children and higher in older children and adolescents, especially among those with obesity. The combined rates of prehypertension and HTN render high BP a very common chronic condition of children and adolescents.

Childhood HTN also has some striking similarities to HTN in adults. Severe untreated HTN in children has as poor an outcome as it does in adults.[3] Children with essential HTN can express the same risk factors for CVD as adults, and children with HTN can benefit from interventions to control BP.[4] An important aspect in the management of high BP in the young is to determine when elevated BP is a sign of an underlying disease, as with secondary HTN, and when elevated BP in childhood is an early expression of primary (essential) HTN.

Definition of HTN in Childhood

There is a progressive normal rise in the BP level with increasing age throughout childhood. The increase in BP level with increasing age is concurrent with the normal age-related increase in height and weight throughout childhood. Thus, there is a consistent relationship of BP with body size in childhood, and there is a normal upward shift in BP with growth. A gender difference in BP distribution emerges in adolescence that is concurrent with a gender difference in height.

The current definition of HTN in children and adolescents is systolic and/ or diastolic BP that, on repeated measurement, is equal to or greater than the 95th percentile for age, sex, and height.[4] The severity of HTN is staged. Stage 1 HTN is systolic or diastolic BP that is between the 95th percentile and 5 mm Hg above the 99th percentile. Stage 2 HTN is average systolic or diastolic BP that is greater than 5 mm Hg above the 99th percentile for age, sex, and height. Prehypertension in children is defined as systolic or diastolic BP that is between the 90th and 95th percentile for age, sex, and height. Because the BP level at the 90th percentile is greater than 120/80 mm Hg in some taller adolescents, a BP level that is greater than 120/80 mm Hg but less than the 95th percentile is considered prehypertension in adolescents. Normal BP is systolic and diastolic BP that is less than the 90th percentile for age, sex, and height. Tables that provide the level of BP for the 90th, 95th, and 99th percentile for age, sex, and height for boys and girls can be accessed at www.nhlbi.nih.gov/guidelines/hypertension/child_tbl.htm. In each table, the 50th percentile for systolic and diastolic BP is also provided to denote the midpoint of the BP distribution.

HTN can also occur in newborns. Although the data on normal levels of BP in newborns and very young infants are somewhat limited, the upper 95% confidence limit for a term infant (40 weeks gestation) is 90 mm Hg for systolic BP. BP levels that exceed 90 mm Hg are considered to be hypertensive in a term infant, and by 4 to 6 weeks of age an SBP that exceeds 100 mm Hg is HTN.

Measurement of BP in the Young

Measurement of BP in children and adolescents should be performed in a standardized manner that is similar to the methods used in the development of the BP tables. In an ambulatory clinic setting, the preferred method for BP measurement in children is auscultation with a standard sphygmomanometer.

Correct BP measurement in children requires the use of a cuff that is appropriate for the size of the child's upper arm. A technique that can be used to select a BP cuff of appropriate size is to select a cuff that has a bladder width that is approximately 40% of the arm circumference midway between the olecranon and the acromion. This will usually be a cuff bladder that will cover 80% to 100% of the circumference of the arm. The equipment necessary to measure BP in children 3 years of age through adolescence includes three pediatric cuffs of different sizes, as well as a standard adult cuff, an oversized cuff, and a thigh cuff for leg BP measurements. The latter two cuffs may be needed for obese adolescents.

BP measurement in children should be conducted in a quiet and comfortable environment after 3 to 5 minutes of rest. With the exception of acute illness, the BP should be measured with the child in the seated position with the arm supported at heart level. It is preferable that the child has his or her feet on the floor while the BP is measured rather than dangling from an exam table. Over-inflation of the cuff should be avoided due to discomfort, particularly in younger children. The BP should be measured and recorded at least twice on each measurement occasion.

Elevated BP measurements in a child or adolescent should be confirmed on repeated visits to verify a diagnosis of HTN in a child. A more accurate characterization of an individual's BP level is an average of multiple BP measurements taken for weeks or months. An exception to this guideline for asymptomatic generally well children would be situations in which the child is symptomatic or has profoundly elevated BP. Automated devices to measure BP in children are being used with increasing frequency. Situations in which use of an automated devices is acceptable include BP measurement in newborn and young infants in whom auscultation is difficult, as well as in an intensive care setting, where frequent BP measurement is necessary. The reliability of these instruments in an ambulatory clinical setting is less clear because of the need for frequent calibration of the instruments and the current lack of established reference standards.

Ambulatory BP monitoring for 24 hours, used in the evaluation of adults with HTN, can also be used in older children and adolescents. Some population standards for ambulatory BP values in children and adolescents are now available, and there are situations in which this information can be quite helpful.[5] Ambulatory BP measurement can be used to verify the diagnosis of HTN, to detect white coat HTN, to determine the need for pharmacologic therapy, and to assess the effectiveness of therapeutic interventions. In children or adolescents, the appropriate cuff size should be used and the appropriate childhood BP cut-points should be used to interpret the results.

Causes of HTN in the Young

Secondary HTN

Underlying causes of HTN, or secondary HTN due to underlying renal or endocrine disorders, occur relatively more frequently in hypertensive children than in hypertensive adults. The rates of secondary HTN in the young vary according to the age and severity of HTN. Young children, less than 12 years of age, with sustained stage 2 HTN are more likely to have a secondary cause for the HTN. The degree of HTN is also an important clue, as severe BP elevation in a young child is most likely to be due to an underlying abnormality. Children and adolescents with stage 2 HTN should have a careful evaluation for a possible cause of the HTN and also for evidence of target-organ damage from the HTN. Although the list of conditions that can cause HTN in the young is quite long, the majority of the identifiable causes of HTN in the young are related to renal disorders. Table 6d.1 provides a list of underlying causes for chronic HTN in the young.

For children up to 10 years of age, the leading causes of HTN are renal parenchymal diseases, coarctation of the aorta, and renal artery stenosis. Coarctation of the aorta, a congenital cardiac anomaly that can be missed in infants and toddlers, should be considered in a hypertensive child. In later childhood, essential HTN can also be detected. Diseases that cause acute HTN include post-infectious glomerulonephritis and hemolytic uremic syndrome. Hemolytic uremic syndrome may cause permanent renal scarring, leading to chronic HTN.

In adolescence the most common cause of HTN is essential HTN. The secondary causes of HTN that are detected most frequently in adolescents are renal parenchymal diseases, such as chronic pyelonephritis and several types of chronic glomerulonephritis. Adolescent behaviors that may contribute to high BP are illicit substance use, especially cocaine and amphetamine-related compounds. Other substances that have been associated with high BP in adolescents include appetite suppressants (both prescription and over-the-counter remedies), oral contraceptives, excessive alcohol intake, and use of anabolic steroids for body building.

Essential HTN

The concept that essential HTN has its roots in childhood can be inferred from BP tracking data, which demonstrate that children with elevated BPs will

Table 6d.1 Secondary Causes of HTN	
Renal	*Syndromes*
Chronic glomerulonephritis	Alport syndrome (renal)
Interstitial nephritis	Williams (renovascular lesions)
Collagen vascular diseases	Turner (coarctation or renovascular)
Reflux nephropathy	Tuberous sclerosis (cystic renal)
Polycystic kidney disease	Neurofibromatosis (renovascular)
Medullary cystic disease	Adrenogenital syndromes
Hydronephrosis	Liddle syndrome
Hypoplastic/dysplastic kidney	*Drugs*
Vascular	Corticosteroids
Coarctation of aorta	Alcohol
Renal artery stenosis	Appetite suppressants
Takayasu arteritis	Anabolic steroids
Endocrine	Oral contraceptives
Hyperthyroidism	Nicotine
Pheochromocytoma	
Primary aldosteronism	

continue to have elevated BPs as adults. Classic risk factors for HTN such as overweight and a positive family history of HTN or CVD are commonly present. Using echocardiography, and appropriate childhood reference values for cardiac structure, LV hypertrophy has been reported in 30% to 40% of children and adolescents with HTN.[6] Longitudinal data are now becoming available that demonstrate a direct link between risk factors in childhood, including BP levels, with evidence of target-organ injury including greater intima-media thickness of carotid arteries.[7] Essential HTN in childhood should be considered an early phase of a chronic disease.

Children and adolescents with essential HTN generally demonstrate several clinical characteristics or associated risk factors. The degree of BP elevation is generally mild, approximating the 95th percentile, and there is often considerable variability in BP over time. The cluster of mild BP elevation, a positive family history of HTN, and obesity is a typical pattern in children and adolescents with essential HTN. The prevalence of childhood obesity has more than doubled in the past 20 years,[8] with a parallel increase in childhood BP level.[9] Metabolic syndrome can also be identified in children, especially among those with obesity and mild BP elevation.[10]

Evaluation of HTN in Children and Adolescents

Children with sustained HTN (BP >95th percentile) require a medical evaluation. The extent of the diagnostic evaluation is determined by the type of HTN that is suspected. When a secondary cause is considered, a more extensive evaluation may be necessary. On the other hand, when the patient's elevated

BP is more likely to be an early expression of essential HTN, fewer diagnostic studies may be needed. Currently, the recommendations for evaluation of HTN in children include (1) evaluation for an identifiable cause; (2) evaluation for comorbidity; and (3) evaluation for target-organ damage.[4]

The medical history and physical examination are keys in determining whether the characteristics of a patient's presentation indicate essential HTN or reflect a secondary, and potentially correctable, cause. Any pediatric patient who is hypertensive and is not growing normally should also undergo an evaluation for secondary causes. A sudden onset of elevated BP in a previously normotensive child should always prompt a search for secondary causes. Absence of a positive family history of HTN should increase the level of suspicion for an underlying disorder. Older children and adolescents with characteristics suggestive of essential HTN (mild BP elevation, obesity, family history of HTN) require less extensive evaluation. Alternatively, it is the children with early expression of essential HTN who may have associated comorbidities, particularly those who are obese. The associated comorbidities include dyslipidemia, sleep apnea, and impaired fasting glucose.

Basic laboratory studies include standard blood chemistries, urinalysis, and a renal ultrasound. An evaluation for the presence of comorbidity includes fasting plasma lipids for dyslipidemia and a sleep history to screen for sleep apnea; if there is a positive family history of diabetes, additional testing of glucose tolerance may be indicated. Measurement of LV mass by echocardiography is a sensitive method to detect target-organ damage in children and adolescents.

Treatment of HTN in Children and Adolescents

Children and adolescents with stage 1 or mild elevation of BP, and without target-organ damage, should begin treatment with nonpharmacologic interventions including weight reduction if overweight or obese, exercise, and diet modifications. Participation in sports should be encouraged as long as BP is under reasonable control, regular monitoring of BP occurs, and cardiac conditions have been excluded. Because the usual dietary intake of sodium for most children and adolescents in the United States far exceeds nutrient requirements, it is reasonable to reduce sodium intake by decreasing fast-food consumption. Alternatively, diets rich in fresh fruits, fiber, and low-fat dairy should be encouraged.[4]

Pharmacologic therapy is indicated if nonpharmacologic approaches are unsuccessful, or when a child is symptomatic and has severe HTN or target-organ damage. Children with diabetes mellitus or chronic kidney disease may achieve renal protective benefits from BP reduction. For children with these disorders it is reasonable to use pharmacologic therapy to lower BP to a level that is below the 90th percentile for age, sex, and height. The choice of antihypertensive medication must be individualized and depends upon the child's age, the etiology of the HTN, the degree of BP elevation, adverse effects, and concomitant medical conditions. Tables that contain dosing information on antihypertensive drugs that have pediatric label information can be accessed at www.nhlbi.nih.gov/guidelines/HTN/child_tbl.htm.[4]

Summary

Due to the rising rates of childhood obesity, the expression of essential HTN in childhood is increasing. Despite this trend, the possibility of secondary HTN should be considered in a child with documented HTN. Children with suspected secondary HTN may require a more extensive evaluation compared to children and adolescents expressing characteristics of essential HTN. Whether the HTN is determined to be secondary or essential, these children require careful monitoring, interventions to control the BP, and long-term follow-up. Considering the long-term morbidity and mortality associated with essential HTN, interventions, including preventive interventions, which focus on BP control beginning in youth, are needed.

References

1. Hansen ML, Gunn PW, Kaelber DC. Underdiagnosis of hypertension in children and adolescents. *JAMA* 2007;298:874–879.

2. McNiece KL, Poffenbarger TS, Turner JL, Franco KD, Sorof JM, Portman RJ. Prevalence of hypertension and pre-hypertension among adolescents. *J Pediatr* 2007;150:640–644.

3. Still JL, Cottom D. Severe hypertension in childhood. *Arch Dis Child* 1967;42:34–39.

4. National High Blood Pressure Education Program Working Group on High Blood Pressure in Children and Adolescents. The Fourth Report on the Diagnosis, Evaluation and Treatment of High Blood Pressure in Children and Adolescents. *Pediatrics* 2004;114:555–576.

5. Urbina E, Alpert B, Flynn J, et al. Ambulatory blood pressure monitoring in children and adolescents: recommendations for standard assessment: a scientific statement from the American Heart Association Atherosclerosis, Hypertension, and Obesity in Youth Committee of the Council on Cardiovascular Disease in the Young and the Council for High Blood Pressure Research. *Hypertension* 2008;52:433–451.

6. Daniels SR, Loggie JM, Hhoury P, Kimball TR. Left ventricular geometry and severe left ventricular hypertrophy in children and adolescents with essential hypertension. *Circulation* 1998;97:1907–1911.

7. Falkner B, Lurbe E, Schaefer F. High blood pressure in children: Need for improved identification, management and health policy. *J Clin Hypertens* 2010;12:261–276.

8. Ogden CL, Flegal KM, Carroll MD, Johnson CL. Prevalence and trends in overweight among US children and adolescents, 1999–2000. *JAMA* 2002;288:1728–1732.

9. Munter P, He J, Cutler JA, et al. Trends in blood pressure among children and adolescents. *JAMA* 2004;291:2107–2113.

10. Boyd GS, Koenigsberg J, Falkner B, Gidding S, Hassink S. Effect of obesity and high blood pressure on plasma lipid levels in children and adolescents. *Pediatrics* 2005;116:442–446.

e. Obesity and the Metabolic Syndrome

Amgad N. Makaryus, MD and Samy I. McFarlane, MD, MPH

Obesity and the associated metabolic syndrome are rapidly emerging as the epidemics of the 21st century. The literature demonstrates a relationship between HTN, type 2 diabetes mellitus, and several vascular and metabolic abnormalities that are components of the metabolic syndrome. The latest reported statistics show that HTN (defined as untreated SBP of 140 mm Hg or higher, or DBP of 90 mm Hg or higher, or taking antihypertensive medication; or being told at least twice by a physician or other health professional that you have HTN) affects over 74 million Americans (35,700,000 males, 38,800,000 females).[1,2] Of those people with HTN, 77.6% were aware of their condition, and of all people with high BP, 67.9% were under current treatment but 55.9% did not have it controlled. Also, the World Health Organization projects that by the year 2025, more than 5% of the world's population (~300 million people) will suffer from diabetes.[1,2]

HTN associated with the metabolic syndrome has certain pathophysiologic characteristics that provide clinical challenges as well as opportunities for successful therapeutic intervention. The components of the metabolic syndrome, which include insulin resistance/hyperinsulinemia, central obesity, dyslipidemia, HTN, microalbuminuria, increased inflammation, and oxidative stress, are the culprit constellation of factors that need to be targeted in the management of these patients. Further behind-the-scenes pathophysiologic dysregulatory processes (such as tissue activation of the RAAS leading to endothelial dysfunction, microalbuminuria, insulin resistance) are the underlying mechanisms for this constellation. Better understanding of these processes supports the now-emerging notion that HTN in these obese patients with the metabolic syndrome is not only a vascular disease but a metabolic one as well, and therefore opens up many avenues for the treatment of this patient population.[3,4]

Epidemiology of HTN in Diabetes and the Metabolic Syndrome

The prevalence of HTN is expected to increase in the next 25 years from 26.5% in the year 2000 to 29.2% in the year 2025. Specifically, the incidence of HTN in patients with type 2 diabetes is approximately two times higher than in those without diabetes. Further, the prevalence of HTN is particularly high in obese subjects, and it increases with age. Because the prevalence of type 2 diabetes is high in obese subjects and it increases with age, the coexistence of diabetes and HTN is particularly high in obese and/or elderly patients. This coexistence of diabetes and HTN in the same patient has profound effects on the CV system, and BP control in these patients is challenging and largely suboptimal. The coexistence of multiple CV risk factors requires treatment on multiple levels, and the treating provider needs to recognize the varied clinical characteristics underlying these factors.[5]

Characteristic Clinical Features and Pathophysiology of HTN Associated with Obesity and the Metabolic Syndrome

The metabolic syndrome is defined as a constellation of metabolic lipid and non-lipid risk factors predisposing to CVD and chronic kidney disease (CKD). Insulin resistance contributes to the pathogenesis of HTN through a number of abnormalities in insulin signaling, and is associated with CV and metabolic derangements. Currently microalbuminuria is recognized as not only a component of the cardiometabolic syndrome, but also as an early marker. Salt sensitivity is present in these patients and leads to a direct volume expansion and increase in BP, specifically systolic HTN, through activation of the RAAS (Table 6e.1).

Insulin Resistance

Insulin resistance is a physiologic condition where insulin becomes less effective at lowering blood sugar levels. The resulting increase in blood glucose may raise levels outside the normal range and cause adverse effects. The given concentration of insulin produces a less-than-expected biologic effect. The syndromes of insulin resistance actually make up a broad clinical spectrum, which includes obesity, glucose intolerance, and diabetes.[6]

In insulin resistance, clinical heterogeneity can be explained on a biochemical basis. Insulin binds and acts mainly through the insulin receptor and also acts via the insulin-like growth factor-1 (IGF-1) receptor; cellular actions of insulin involve a wide variety of effects on post-receptor signaling pathways within target cells. Ambient insulin levels, various physiologic and disease states, and drugs regulate insulin receptor concentration or affinity. The mechanisms

Table 6e.1 Clinical and Pathophysiologic Characteristics of HTN Associated with Diabetes and the Metabolic Syndrome
1. Insulin resistance
2. RAAS stimulation
3. Microalbuminuria
4. Salt sensitivity
5. Volume expansion
6. Systolic hypertension
7. Orthostatic hypotension

responsible for insulin resistance syndromes include genetic or primary target cell defects, autoantibodies to insulin, and accelerated insulin degradation.[6,7]

Patients with obesity have a decreased number of receptors and further post-receptor failure to activate factors is present. While adiposity and insulin resistance are related, each may make its own independent and different contribution to increasing the risk of CVD. Insulin resistance plays a major pathogenic role in the development of the metabolic syndrome through various derangements, such as hyperinsulinemia, type 2 diabetes or glucose intolerance, central obesity, HTN, dyslipidemia, and hypercoagulability.[6,7]

Insulin resistance and the compensatory hyperinsulinemia are associated with an increased CVD risk, especially through endothelial dysfunction, which is a prominent feature of the insulin resistance syndrome. Type 2 diabetes is characterized by increased hepatic glucose output, increased peripheral resistance to insulin's action, and impaired insulin secretion. In skeletal muscle, various abnormalities, including defective glucose transport, lead to insulin resistance and the resulting effects.[6,7]

Microalbuminuria

Microalbuminuria (defined as urinary albumin excretion of 30 to 300 mg/24 hours) is one of the earliest markers of diabetic nephropathy. Microalbuminuria may progress over a span of a number of years to overt nephropathy and eventually renal failure requiring dialysis. Studies have shown that microalbuminuria is reversible with interventions to tightly control blood sugar and BP.[8,9]

Both HTN and nephropathy appear to exacerbate each other. Elevated SBP is a significant determining factor in the progression of microalbuminuria.[10,11] There is an increasing evidence that microalbuminuria is an integral component of the metabolic syndrome associated with HTN.[9,10] This concept is important to consider in selecting the pharmacologic therapy for HTN in patients with diabetes, where medications that decrease both proteinuria and BP such as ACE inhibitors and ARBs have evolved as increasingly important tools in reducing the progression of nephropathy in these patients.[9,12]

Salt Sensitivity and Volume Expansion

Salt sensitivity is defined as an increase in BP in response to increased sodium ingestion and/or a decrease in BP when sodium intake is reduced, with the degree of change exceeding that attributed to directionally appropriate random BP variation. This sensitivity results from alterations in renal function that require higher arterial pressure to maintain "steady-state" homeostasis, and results in volume expansion to reach a higher BP level in order to excrete a given amount of dietary sodium.[13,14]

It is essential to realize that intricate to the development of HTN in patients are alterations in sodium balance and extracellular fluid volume with their heterogeneous effects on BP. Increased salt intake does not necessarily raise BP in all hypertensive subjects. Further, sensitivity to dietary salt intake is greatest in the elderly; those with diabetes, obesity, renal insufficiency, or low renin status;

and African-Americans. Salt sensitivity in normotensive subjects is associated with a greater age-related increase in BP. Since the prevalence of both diabetes and salt sensitivity increases with age, it is particularly important to consider this in management of HTN in these patients.[13–15]

Systolic HTN

Systolic HTN is caused by the progression of atherosclerosis in patients causing the larger arteries to lose elasticity and become rigid and the SBP to increase disproportionately because the arterial system is incapable of expansion for any given volume of blood ejected from the LV. Although this tends to occur at older ages, in patients with diabetes and the metabolic syndrome it is more common and occurs at a relatively younger age.[16]

Orthostatic Hypotension

Orthostatic hypotension is caused by the pooling of blood in dependent veins during rising from a recumbent position. This generally leads to a decrease in stroke volume and SBP with concomitant increase in systemic vascular resistance, DBP, and heart rate. In the presence of autonomic dysfunction, especially in patients with diabetes, excessive venous pooling can cause immediate or delayed orthostatic hypotension that might cause reduction in cerebral blood flow, leading to intermittent lightheadedness, fatigue, unsteady gait, and syncope. This hypotension has several diagnostic and therapeutic implications, such as discontinuation of diuretic therapy and volume repletion. Furthermore, doses of all antihypertensive agents must be titrated more carefully in patients with diabetes, who have a greater propensity for orthostatic hypotension while having high supine BPs.[17]

Stimulation of RAAS

The agent angiotensin II, which is the central potentiator in the RAAS, elevates BP by a variety of mechanisms, including direct vasoconstriction, potentiation of sympathetic nervous system activity at both central and peripheral levels, stimulation of aldosterone synthesis and release with consequent sodium and fluid retention by the kidney, and stimulation of arginine vasopressin release. Angiotensin II also has a variety of actions that damage blood vessels directly. It stimulates NADH and NADPH activity, raising the oxidative potential of vascular tissue. It stimulates leukocyte adhesion to the site of injury and favors superoxide and peroxynitrite formation and proliferation and migration of various cell types toward the luminal site of injury. The series of events that follow cause cellular components of the arterial wall to transform their phenotypes, resulting in neointimal proliferation of atherosclerotic plaque and fibrous plaque. Angiotensin II also has an effect on the thrombotic cascade by its stimulation of synthesis of the antithrombolytic agent, PAI-1, thereby predisposing to atherosclerosis and thromboembolic events.[18]

Increases in systemic RAAS activity enhance the insulin-resistant state through its inhibitory effects on insulin signaling pathway (Fig. 6e.1). Furthermore, it has been postulated that increased free fatty acids (FFAs), through their effects on

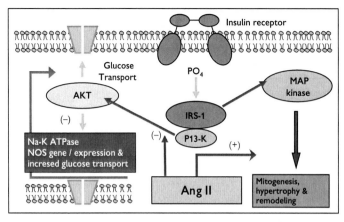

Figure 6e.1 By inhibiting the insulin signaling pathway, angiotensin II contributes to the insulin-resistant state associated with HTN in people with diabetes.

the liver, may contribute to the elevated aldosterone levels in the insulin resistance state. Further, emerging evidence demonstrates that angiotensin II, ACE levels, and plasma renin activity correlate with body mass index (BMI).[19]

Management of HTN in the Obese Population with Metabolic Syndrome

The goal of treating HTN in patients with diabetes and the metabolic syndrome is to prevent the associated macrovascular and microvascular morbidity and mortality. The metabolic syndrome is considered a coronary disease equivalent and, therefore, necessitates an aggressive approach similar to that for patients with CAD.

For a long time, all major guidelines, including those of the American Heart Association and the Seventh Report of the Joint National Committee on Prevention, Detection, Evaluation, and Treatment of High BP, have argued for more aggressive treatment goals. Specifically, in those with diabetes, CAD, or kidney disease, the recommendation is to lower BP to levels below 130/80 mm Hg.[20] These recommendations for lower BP goals in these specific groups were derived from retrospective data analyses. However, the goal of less than 130/80 mm Hg has not been definitively shown as the target. In the meta-analyses of all clinical trials to date that demonstrate the beneficial effect on stroke and coronary disease of reducing BP, none has achieved a mean BP goal of less than 130/80 mm Hg.[21] In trials such as the United Kingdom Prospective Diabetes Study (UKPDS)[22] and the Hypertension Optimal Treatment (HOT) trial,[23] the SBP was more than 10 mm Hg higher than this lower goal. However, despite the lack of reaching the BP goal, a benefit still occurred in terms of CVD reduction. What seems to be the case from these trials is that decreasing BP decreases events, but the level of cutoff does not seem to be the target.

The recently published Action to Control Cardiovascular Risk in Diabetes (ACCORD) BP trial,[24] studied a total of 4,733 participants with type 2 diabetes and randomly assigned them to intensive therapy, targeting an SBP of less than 120 mm Hg, or standard therapy, targeting an SBP of less than 140 mm Hg. The primary composite outcome over a mean follow-up of 4.7 years was nonfatal MI, nonfatal stroke, or death from CV causes. The annual rate of the primary outcome was 1.87% in the intensive-therapy group and 2.09% in the standard-therapy group (hazard ratio with intensive therapy, 0.88; 95% confidence interval [CI], 0.73–1.06; $p = 0.20$). The annual rates of death from any cause were 1.28% and 1.19% in the two groups, respectively (hazard ratio, 1.07; 95% CI, 0.85–1.35; $p = 0.55$). This shows that in patients with type 2 diabetes at high risk for CV events, targeting an SBP of less than 120 mm Hg, as compared with less than 140 mm Hg, did not reduce the rate of a composite outcome of fatal and nonfatal major CV events.[24] Despite these findings, consensus still dictates that a multitargeted program consisting of pharmacologic and nonpharmacologic measures to control various underlying risk factors should be employed in all patients, and that the pharmacologic arm of the approach generally requires the use of multiple medications for adequate effect.

Lifestyle Interventions

Lifestyle modification is the basis for any treatment regimen in these patients. Weight loss should be encouraged for all overweight patients; even moderate weight loss with proper diet can improve BP. Even a modest weight loss, up to 5% to 10% of initial body weight, may reduce the CVD risk substantially. In the Diabetes Prevention Program, a lifestyle intervention including diet and regular exercise achieving weight reduction by 5% to 7% of initial body weight reduced the likelihood of diabetes by 58% compared to 38% with metformin. The DASH diet lowers both BP and low-density lipoprotein (LDL) cholesterol.[25–27] Alcohol consumption should be limited to two drinks or fewer per day. All adults should be encouraged to participate in regular, moderately intense (40% to 60% of maximal oxygen consumption) physical activity for 50 to 60 minutes three or four times per week. Regular physical activity reduces very-low-density lipoprotein (VLDL) levels, raises high-density lipoprotein (HDL) cholesterol, and in some persons lowers LDL levels. It can also lower BP, reduce insulin resistance, and favorably influence CV function.[25–27] While nonpharmacologic lifestyle intervention measures are essential, it is now recognized that pharmacologic therapy should often be instituted concomitantly due to the importance of drug therapy in reducing CVD in this high-risk group.

Antihypertensive Therapy

While targets for BP lowering in these patients are currently under question due to results of the ACCORD trial,[24] one thing that is certain is that lowering BP is important to decrease morbidity and mortality in these patients. This is agreed upon because of the association of elevated BP with CV risk, which is amplified in patients with type 2 diabetes, who have roughly a doubling of absolute risk compared with patients without type 2 diabetes at each SBP level.[28] It is estimated that in patients with stage 1 HTN (SBP 140 to 159 mm Hg and/or DBP 90 to 99 mm Hg) and additional CVD risk factors, achieving a sustained 12-mm Hg decrease in SBP for 10 years will prevent 1 death for every 11 patients treated. In the presence of CVD or target-organ damage, only 9 patients would require this BP reduction to prevent a death.[29]

Several trials have demonstrated the benefit of BP control in patients with type 2 diabetes. This control and the resulting benefit are accomplished with a combination of diuretics and other agents. Inclusion of agents that target the RAAS in the treatment regimen has particular benefits in patients with type 2 diabetes and the metabolic syndrome, and evidence suggests that these benefits are due to both BP-dependent and -independent effects. Recent reviews suggest that more than 65% of people with type 2 diabetes and HTN will require at least two different antihypertensive medications to achieve BP reduction.[10,30] Thiazide diuretics, beta-blockers, ACE inhibitors, ARBs, and CCBs are beneficial in reducing CVD and stroke incidence in patients with type 2 diabetes.[30–34]

Diuretics

Diuretics have long been considered the first-line and basic treatment strategy for most patients with HTN. Specifically, thiazide-type diuretics have been the basis of antihypertensive therapy in most outcome trials. In these trials, including the Antihypertensive and Lipid-Lowering Treatment to Prevent Heart Attack Trial (ALLHAT),[32] diuretics have shown great ability in preventing the CV complications of HTN. Diuretics enhance the antihypertensive efficacy of multiple-drug regimens and are considered integral in these regimens. However, thiazide diuretics should still be used with some caution, especially in patients who have gout or who have a history of significant hyponatremia, and even in diabetics, as they have been implicated in worsening of insulin resistance and increasing the risk of type 2 diabetes.[32]

ACE Inhibitors

ACE inhibitors are an integral component of any antihypertensive regimen in patients with type 2 diabetes and the metabolic syndrome, as these agents have been demonstrated to reduce CVD[34–36] and CKD.[32,33] The use of the ACE inhibitor ramipril was associated with a significant 25% risk reduction in MI, stroke, or CV death after a median follow-up of 4.5 years in the 3,577 patients with type 2 diabetes in the Heart Outcomes Prevention Evaluation (HOPE) trial. This benefit was independent of the BP-lowering effect. In the MICRO-HOPE sub-study, ramipril treatment was associated with a decreased risk of development of overt nephropathy in patients with type 2 diabetes.[37] Other ACE inhibitors, for example captopril, also markedly lowered the risk for fatal and nonfatal MI, stroke, and CV deaths compared with the conventional therapy group.[38]

ACE inhibitors are also known to decrease intraglomerular pressure and glomerular membrane permeability to albumin, therefore contributing to decreases in microalbuminuria and overt proteinuria. The Bergamo Nephrologic Diabetes Complications Trial (BENEDICT) study included 1,204 patients with type 2 diabetes and HTN. At the beginning of the study, none of the patients had any signs of kidney disease. Subjects were randomly assigned to receive at least 3 years of treatment with trandolapril (2 mg/day) plus verapamil (sustained-release formulation, 180 mg/day), trandolapril alone (2 mg/day), verapamil alone (sustained-release formulation, 240 mg/day), or placebo. The target BP was 120/80 mm Hg. The primary endpoint was the development of persistent microalbuminuria (overnight albumin excretion of at least 20 mcg/min at two consecutive visits). After an average of 3.5 years, patients who had good BP control, regardless of which treatment they received, had lower rates of microalbuminuria. Patients taking the combination treatment trandolapril plus verapamil and trandolapril alone had a delayed onset of microalbuminuria by factors of 2.6 and 2.1, respectively. Therefore, taking an ACE inhibitor, alone or as part of the combination treatment, provided further protection against diabetic kidney disease. This was also the case for patients whose BP remained high: as long as they were taking an ACE inhibitor, their microalbuminuria risk was similar to that of patients whose BP was well controlled.[39]

Certain patients may not tolerate an ACE inhibitor, either because of specific side effects from therapy or because of absolute contraindications. If a persistent cough secondary to the ACE inhibitor is intolerable and precludes its further use, then use of an ARB appears appropriate. Other complications of ACE inhibitor therapy, particularly in patients with diabetes, may be the progression of renal functional impairment and/or hyperkalemia. In these patients, a CCB may be appropriate.[34]

ARBs

The antihypertensive efficacy of ARBs is equivalent to that of ACE inhibitors, and they have been shown to have an improved side-effect profile. The decreased side-effect profile of ARBs in comparison to ACE inhibitors may clinically translate into improved compliance. Similar to ACE inhibitors, ARBs offer additional benefits in patients with type 2 diabetes.

The Losartan Intervention For Endpoint Reduction in HTN (LIFE) trial of losartan versus atenolol showed that the use of losartan leads to a significant 13% reduction in CV death, a 13% reduction in MI, and a 25% risk reduction of stroke. The subset of patients with type 2 diabetes in this study had an even more significant reduction (24%) in the primary endpoint, as well as in CV mortality (37%) and total mortality (39%) when compared to atenolol.[40] The Reduction of Endpoints in NIDDM with Angiotensin II Antagonist Losartan (RENAAL) trial showed that ARBs reduce proteinuria and the time to creatinine doubling *and* slow the progression of renal disease.[41] In addition, the Irbesartan in Microalbuminiria (IRMA) II trial supported the use of ARBs in reduction in progression to nephropathy.[42] These trials again support the beneficial effects of ARBs on nephropathy as independent of the changes in BP.

Lipid-Lowering Therapy

Dyslipidemia is integral in the pathophysiology of the MS and is typically characterized by high concentrations of triglycerides; the presence of small, dense, LDL particles; and low concentrations of HDL cholesterol. Numerous trials have shown the benefit of using statins in patients with and without diabetes. In the Heart Protection Study (HPS), the benefit of LDL-cholesterol reduction with simvastatin was evaluated in a high-risk patient population with a broad range of cholesterol levels. Treatment with simvastatin was associated with a significant reduction in mortality (12.9% vs. 14.7% in the placebo group), which was primarily due to a reduction in CV mortality. LDL cholesterol reduction therefore can reduce the CV risk in patients with type 2 diabetes, regardless of their baseline LDL cholesterol level.[43] Evidence from the Scandinavian Simvastatin Survival Study (4S) study demonstrated that simvastatin significantly reduced the primary endpoint of total mortality and the secondary endpoint of major coronary events by 30% and 34%, respectively, versus placebo. These trials and numerous others show the need to make anti-hyperlipidemia therapy an essential component of the treatment armamentarium in these patients.[44]

Conclusion

The association and interrelationship of HTN and diabetes in the metabolic syndrome is complex and encompasses many interactive dysregulatory systems that all contribute to increased CV and renal risk. The interrelationship encompasses not only vascular and hemodynamic changes, but also numerous complex metabolic abnormalities that collectively constitute the metabolic syndrome in obese patients. This constellation of derangements, including insulin resistance/hyperinsulinemia and obesity, promote a chronic low-grade inflammatory state that characterizes dysfunctional adipose tissue, activation of the RAAS, and oxidative stress resulting in endothelial dysfunction, microalbuminuria, and ultimately increased CVD risk. Aggressive targeting of these physiologic derangements through application of targeted and validated treatment approaches is the way to decrease morbidity and mortality in these patients.

References

1. Lloyd-Jones D, Adams RJ, Brown TM, Carnethon M, Dai S, De Simone G, Ferguson TB, Ford E, Furie K, Gillespie C, Go A, Greenlund K, Haase N, Hailpern S, Ho PM, Howard V, Kissela B, Kittner S, Lackland D, Lisabeth L, Marelli A, McDermott MM, Meigs J, Mozaffarian D, Mussolino M, Nichol G, Roger VL, Rosamond W, Sacco R, Sorlie P, Stafford R, Thom T, Wasserthiel-Smoller S, Wong ND, Wylie-Rosett J. American Heart Association Statistics Committee and Stroke Statistics Subcommittee. Executive summary: heart disease and stroke statistics—2010 update: a report from the American Heart Association. *Circulation* 2010;121(7):948–954.

2. Heron MP, Hoyert DL, Murphy SL, Xu JQ, Kochanek KD, Tejada-Vera B. Final data for 2006. *National Vital Statistics Reports*; vol. 57, no. 14. Hyattsville, MD: National Center for Health Statistics, 2009.

3. Makaryus AN, Akhrass P, McFarlane SI. Treatment of hypertension in metabolic syndrome: implications of recent clinical trials. *Curr Diab Rep* 2009;9(3):229–237.

4. Ismail H, Mitchell R, McFarlane SI, Makaryus AN. Pleiotropic effects of inhibitors of the RAAS in the diabetic population: above and beyond blood pressure lowering. *Curr Diab Rep* 2010;10(1):32–36.

5. Grossman E, Messerli FH. Hypertension and diabetes. *Adv Cardiol* 2008; 45:82–106.

6. Reaven G, Abbasi F, McLaughlin T. Obesity, insulin resistance, and cardiovascular disease. *Recent Prog Horm Res* 2004;59:207–223.

7. Reaven GM. Pathophysiology of insulin resistance in human disease. *Physiol Rev* 1995;75(3):473–486.

8. Ismail H, Mitchell R, McFarlane SI, Makaryus AN. Pleiotropic effects of inhibitors of the RAAS in the diabetic population: above and beyond blood pressure lowering. *Curr Diab Rep* 2010;10(1):32–36.

9. Tagle R, Acevedo M, Vidt DG. Microalbuminuria: is it a valid predictor of cardiovascular risk? *Cleve Clin J Med* 2003;70:255–261.

10. SHEP Cooperative Research Group. Prevention of stroke by antihypertensive drug treatment in older persons with isolated systolic hypertension. Final results of the Systolic Hypertension in the Elderly Program (SHEP). *JAMA* 1991;265:3255–3264.

11. Dahlof B, Devereux RB, Kjeldsen SE, et al. Cardiovascular morbidity and mortality in the Losartan Intervention For Endpoint reduction in hypertension study (LIFE): a randomised trial against atenolol. *Lancet* 2002;359:995–1003.

12. Makaryus AN, Akhrass P, McFarlane SI. Treatment of hypertension in metabolic syndrome: implications of recent clinical trials. *Curr Diab Rep* 2009;9(3):229–237.

13. Luft F, Weinberger M. Heterogeneous responses to changes in dietary salt intake: The salt sensitivity paradigm. *Am J Clin Nutr* 1997;65(suppl):612S–617S.

14. Sullivan J. Salt sensitivity: Definition, conception, methodology, and long-term issues. *Hypertension* 1991;17(suppl I):I61–I68.

15. Weinberger MH. Salt sensitive human hypertension. *Endocr Res* 1991;17:43–51.

16. Sowers JR, Epstein M, Frohlich ED. Diabetes, hypertension, and cardiovascular disease: an update. *Hypertension* 2001;37:1053–1059.

17. Jacob G, Costa F, Biaggioni I. Spectrum of autonomic cardiovascular neuropathy in diabetes. *Diabetes Care* 2003;26:2174–2180.

18. Bakris GL, Sowers JR, Glies TD, Black HR, Izzo JL Jr, Materson BJ, Oparil S, Weber MA. Treatment of hypertension in patients with diabetes—an update. *J Am Soc Hypertens* 2010;4(2):62–67.

19. Zhang R, Reisin E: Obesity-hypertension; the effects on cardiovascular and renal systems. *Am J Hypertens* 2000;13:1308–1314.

20. Chobanian AV, Bakris GL, Black HR, Cushman WC, Green LA, Izzo JL Jr, Jones DW, Materson BJ, Oparil S, Wright JT Jr, Roccella EJ; National Heart, Lung, and Blood Institute Joint National Committee on Prevention, Detection, Evaluation, and Treatment of High Blood Pressure; National High Blood Pressure Education Program Coordinating Committee: The Seventh Report of the Joint National Committee on Prevention, Detection, Evaluation and Treatment of High Blood Pressure: The JNC 7 Report. *JAMA* 2003;289(19):2560–2571.

21. Hopkins KA, Bakris GL. Lower blood pressure goals in high-risk cardiovascular patients: are they defensible? *Cardiol Clin* 2010;28(3):447–452.

22. Tight blood pressure control and risk of macrovascular and microvascular complications in type 2 diabetes: UKPDS 38. UK Prospective Diabetes Study Group. *BMJ* 1998;317(7160):703–713.

23. Hansson L, Zanchetti A, Carruthers SG, et al. Effects of intensive blood-pressure lowering and low-dose aspirin in patients with hypertension: principal results of the Hypertension Optimal Treatment (HOT) randomised trial. HOT Study Group. *Lancet* 1998;351(9118):1755–1762.

24. ACCORD Study Group, Cushman WC, Evans GW, Byington RP, Goff DC Jr, Grimm RH Jr, Cutler JA, Simons-Morton DG, Basile JN, Corson MA, Probstfield JL, Katz L, Peterson KA, Friedewald WT, Buse JB, Bigger JT, Gerstein HC, Ismail-Beigi F. Effects of intensive blood-pressure control in type 2 diabetes mellitus. *N Engl J Med* 2010;362(17):1575–1585.

25. Sacks FM, Svetkey LP, Vollmer WM, Appel LJ, Bray GA, Harsha D, Obarzanek E, Conlin PR, Miller ER 3rd, Simons-Morton DG, Karanja N, Lin PH. Effects on blood pressure of reduced dietary sodium and the Dietary Approaches to Stop Hypertension (DASH) diet: DASH-Sodium Collaborative Research Group. *N Engl J Med* 2001;344:3–10.

26. Obarzanek E, Sacks FM, Vollmer WM, Bray GA, Miller ER 3rd, Lin PH, Karanja NM, Most-Windhauser MM, Moore TJ, Swain JF, Bales CW, Proschan MA, for the DASH Research Group. Effects on blood lipids of a blood pressure lowering diet: the Dietary Approaches to Stop Hypertension (DASH) Trial. *Am J Clin Nutr* 2001;74:80–89.

27. American Diabetes Association. Treatment of hypertension in adults with diabetes. *Diabetes Care* 2002;25(suppl 1):S71–S73.

28. Stamler J, Vaccaro O, Neaton JD, Wentworth D. Diabetes, other risk factors, and 12-yr cardiovascular mortality for men screened in the Multiple Risk Factor Intervention Trial. *Diabetes Care* 1993;16:434–444.

29. El-Atat F, Aneja A, Mcfarlane S, Sowers J. Obesity and hypertension. *Endocrinol Metab Clin North Am* 2003;32:823–854.

30. Staessen JA, Fagard R, Thijs L, et al. Randomised double-blind comparison of placebo and active treatment for older patients with isolated systolic hypertension. The Systolic Hypertension in Europe (Syst-Eur) Trial Investigators. *Lancet* 1997;350:757–764.

31. Hansson L, Zanchetti A, Carruthers SG, et al. Effects of intensive blood-pressure lowering and low-dose aspirin in patients with hypertension: principal results of the Hypertension Optimal Treatment (HOT) randomised trial. HOT Study Group. *Lancet* 1998;351:1755–1762.

32. The ALLHAT Officers and Coordinators for the ALLHAT Collaborative Research Group. Major outcomes in high-risk hypertensive patients randomized to angiotensin-converting enzyme inhibitor or calcium channel blocker vs. diuretic. *JAMA* 2002;288:2981–2997.

33. UK Prospective Diabetes Study Group. Efficacy of atenolol and captopril in reducing risk of macrovascular and microvascular complications in type 2 diabetes: UKPDS 39. *BMJ* 1998;317:713–720.

34. Makaryus AN, McFarlane SI. Treatment of hypertension in the diabetic patient. *Therapy* 2009;6(4):497–505.

35. Hansson L, Lindholm LH, Niskanen L, Lanke J, Hedner T, Niklason A, Luomanmaki K, Dahlof B, de Faire U, Morlin C, Karlberg BE, Wester PO, Bjork JE. Effect of angiotensin-converting-enzyme inhibition compared with conventional

therapy on cardiovascular morbidity and mortality in hypertension: the Captopril Prevention Project (CAPPP) randomized trial. *Lancet* 1999;353:611–616.

36. Yusuf S, Sleight P, Pogue Bosch J, Davies JR, Dagenais G. Effects of an angiotensin-converting-enzyme inhibitor, ramipril, on cardiovascular events in high-risk patients. The Heart Outcomes Prevention Evaluation Study Investigators. *N Engl J Med* 2000;342:145–153.

37. Heart Outcomes Prevention Evaluation Study Investigators. Effects of ramipril on cardiovascular and microvascular outcomes in people with diabetes mellitus: results of the HOPE study and MICRO-HOPE substudy. *Lancet* 2000;355:253–259.

38. Hansson L, Lindholm LH, Niskanen L, Lanke J, Hedner T, Niklason A, Luomanmaki K, Dahlof B, de Faire U, Morlin C, Karlberg BE, Wester PO, Bjork JE. Effect of angiotensin-converting-enzyme inhibition compared with conventional therapy on cardiovascular morbidity and mortality in hypertension: the Captopril Prevention Project (CAPPP) randomized trial. *Lancet* 1999;353:611–616.

39. Ruggenenti P, Fassi A, Ilieva AP, Bruno S, Iliev IP, Brusegan V, Rubis N, Gherardi G, Arnoldi F, Ganeva M, Ene-Iordache B, Gaspari F, Perna A, Bossi A, Trevisan R, Dodesini AR, Remuzzi G; Bergamo Nephrologic Diabetes Complications Trial (BENEDICT) Investigators. Preventing microalbuminuria in type 2 diabetes. *N Engl J Med* 2004;351(19):1941–1951.

40. Lindholm LH, Ibsen H, Dahlof B, et al. Cardiovascular morbidity and mortality in patients with diabetes in the Losartan Intervention For Endpoint reduction in hypertension study (LIFE): a randomised trial against atenolol. *Lancet* 2002;359:1004–1010.

41. Whaley-Connell A, Sowers JR. Hypertension management in type 2 diabetes and the JNC VII. *Endocrinol Metabol Clin North Am* 2005;34(1):63–75.

42. Parving HH, Lehnert H, Brochner-Mortensen J, Gomis R, Andersen S, Arner P. The effect of irbesartan on the development of diabetic nephropathy in patients with type 2 diabetes. *N Engl J Med* 2001;345(12):870–878.

43. Armitage J, Collins R. Need for large-scale randomised evidence about lowering LDL cholesterol in people with diabetes mellitus: MRC/BHF heart protection study and other major trials MRC/BHF Heart Protection Study. *Heart* 2000;84:357–360.

44. Pyorala K, Ballantyne CM, Gumbiner B, Lee MW, Shah A, Davies MJ, Mitchel YB, Pedersen TR, Kjekshus J, the Scandinavian Simvastatin Survival Study (4S): Reduction of cardiovascular events by simvastatin in nondiabetic coronary heart disease patients with and without the metabolic syndrome: subgroup analyses of the Scandinavian Simvastatin Survival Study (4S). *Diabetes Care* 2004;27:1735–1740.

f. Peripheral Arterial Disease

Asterios Karagiannis, MD, Vasilios G. Athyros, MD,
Konstantinos Tziomalos, MD, PhD, and
Dimitri P. Mikhailidis, MD

A 67-year-old Caucasian man was admitted to the hospital because of a 6-month history of intermittent claudication in both legs. There was a 12-year history of HTN and a 5-year history of type 2 diabetes mellitus. The patient has been smoking 1 pack of cigarettes daily for the past 42 years. His medications comprised irbesartan/hydrochlorothiazide 300/12.5 mg once a day, metformin 850 mg once a day, and atorvastatin 20 mg once a day. On physical examination, BP was 125/80 mm Hg and heart rate 74 was bpm. Both legs showed signs of peripheral arterial disease (PAD), including loss of hair with cold, thin, and dry skin. Pulses in the dorsalis pedis and posterior tibial arteries were not palpable, also suggesting the presence of PAD. The ankle–brachial index (ABI) was 0.76 in the right leg and 0.82 in the left leg. On admission, results of laboratory tests were within the normal range except glucose (178 mg/dL [9.9 mmol/L]) and HbA1c levels (7.4%). The ECG was normal. Digital subtraction angiography revealed severe atherosclerosis involving both external iliac arteries (84% and 90% stenosis in the right and left external iliac artery, respectively) and both superficial femoral arteries (92% and 95% stenosis in the right and left superficial femoral artery, respectively). Percutaneous transluminal angioplasty with stent placement in all affected arteries restored distal blood flow. The patient was advised to quit smoking and to exercise every day. Low-dose aspirin (80 mg) was added and the dose of metformin was increased (850 mg twice a day). The patient is well during a 2-year follow-up period without recurrent symptoms of PAD.

Lower extremity PAD affects a considerable proportion of elderly subjects worldwide. [1-3] The prevalence of PAD varies greatly depending on the population studied, the definition used (symptomatic PAD or not), the diagnostic method, age, sex, and the presence of other vascular risk factors.[1-5] PAD is associated with disability and reduced quality of life as well as with significant morbidity and mortality from CVD.[3,4] PAD represents a strong predictor of MI, stroke, and death from vascular causes.[3,4] Patients with PAD have a six times greater 10-year mortality risk from MI or stroke than subjects without PAD.[3,4] Symptomatic PAD is associated with a 15-fold increase in the 10-year mortality rate.[3,4] The Reduction of Atherothrombosis for Continued Health (REACH) registry, comprising more than 68,000 patients, showed that subjects with documented PAD had higher 1-year CVD event rates (including CVD death, MI, stroke, or hospitalization for atherothrombotic events) than patients with coronary heart disease (CHD) or cerebrovascular disease.[5,6]

Atherosclerosis represents the primary pathogenetic mechanism leading to PAD and is considered a chronic progressive systemic disease of multifactorial etiology.[3] Atherosclerosis can affect the coronary, cerebrovascular, and peripheral vasculature, but the rate of progression can vary among vascular beds.[3] Patients who experience symptoms of ischemia in one vascular bed often have severe atherosclerosis in other vascular beds.[3] Irreversible risk factors contributing to the development of atherosclerosis and PAD are advanced age, male gender, black race, and family history.[1,3,5] Reversible risk factors include HTN, diabetes mellitus, dyslipidemia, and tobacco use.[1,3]

PAD affects approximately 27 million people in North America and Europe and its prevalence increases with age, being 4.3% in subjects under the age of 40, 20% in those over 55, and up to 60% in those older than 85 years.[1-3] Data from the National Health and Nutrition Examination Survey (NHANES) 1999–2000 showed that 24% of individuals older than 40 years with a creatinine clearance below 60 mL/min/1.73 m^2 had an ABI of less than 0.9.[3] Prevalence of symptomatic PAD is only slightly higher among men compared with women, and this difference seems to narrow after the age of 70 years.[3] Epidemiologic studies demonstrated that blacks are disproportionately affected by PAD, with a two- to three-fold increase in risk compared with whites.[3] According to the U.S. Renal Data report, among dialysis patients, the incidence of clinical PAD is 15%.[3] No gene has yet been clearly associated with the development of PAD, but there is increased occurrence of PAD in relatives of patients with intermittent claudication.[3,5]

Smoking is the most important modifiable risk factor for PAD.[1,3] In subjects older than 45 years, the estimated risk of developing PAD is 16-fold higher among smokers.[1,3] Smokers have poorer survival rates than non-smokers and a two-fold increased risk for developing critical limb ischemia leading to amputation.[1,3] The association between smoking and development of PAD is two times stronger than that between smoking and CHD.[1,3] HTN is also strongly associated with PAD, and the coexistence of these diseases substantially increases the risk for CVD.[1,3] The NHANES and the PAD Awareness, Risk, and Treatment: New Resources for Survival (PARTNERS) programs reported that HTN is present in 74% to 92% of patients with PAD.[3] The Framingham Heart Study showed a 2.5- to 4-fold increased risk of claudication in hypertensive patients.[3] In addition, atheromatous renal artery stenosis (RAS) can be the underlying cause of HTN in patients with PAD.[2] After adjustment for age and HTN, RAS incidence was four times higher in patients with three or four peripheral arteries affected.[2] Diabetes also increases the risk for PAD 1.5- to 4-fold.[1,3] Patients with diabetes and PAD may develop neuropathy and impaired wound healing and are at higher risk for ischemic ulceration and gangrene, leading to a higher rate of amputations.[1,3] Dyslipidemia is associated with a two-fold increase in the risk for intermittent claudication.[1,3] The NHANES and the PARTNERS programs reported a 60% to 77% prevalence of dyslipidemia in patients with PAD.[1,3] Elevated levels of C-reactive protein (CRP) indicate the presence of inflammation in the arterial bed and have also been linked to the development of atherosclerosis and PAD.[3]

Despite its considerable prevalence and the high CVD risk, PAD remains underdiagnosed and undertreated.[1,3] Early detection of PAD, particularly in its asymptomatic stage, and aggressive management significantly reduce CVD risk.[3] A detailed medical history should focus on symptoms of claudication, rest pain, impaired ability to walk, and non-healing lower extremity wounds.[3] However, many studies revealed that only 10% to 33% of patients with PAD present with typical claudication symptoms.[1,3,4] Hair loss, thin skin, thick nails, tapering toes, and wounds or ulcers in the legs or feet are signs of prolonged ischemia.[3] Diminished bilateral peripheral pulses, femoral bruits, and prolonged capillary refill time are signs suggestive of PAD.[3]

Patients with suggestive clinical history and physical examination should undergo determination of ABI, a simple, quick, painless, noninvasive, highly reproducible, and accurate test for the diagnosis of PAD.[3,4] Normal ABI values range from 0.90 to 1.30.[3,4] Patients with claudication frequently have an ABI value between 0.50 and 0.85, and values below 0.30 are commonly seen in patients with rest pain or gangrene.[3,4] An ABI of 0.9 or less is associated with increased risk for fatal and nonfatal CHD, stroke, and all-cause mortality.[3,4] It has also been shown that patients with an ABI of 1.40 and up have similar mortality rates to those with an ABI of 0.9 or less.[3,4] High ABI values reflect medial arterial calcification as well as stiffened and incompressible arteries.[3,4] Toe–brachial index (TBI) is more helpful in patients with rigid, calcified, and noncompliant blood vessels (e.g., in those with diabetes or advanced chronic kidney disease [CKD], or those on dialysis).[3,4] A TBI value of 0.80 or higher is considered normal.[3,4] Once the diagnosis of PAD is established, arterial duplex ultrasonography and magnetic resonance arteriography are useful methods to identify the location and severity of arterial disease.[3] A treadmill test is also helpful in diagnosing whether symptoms are due to PAD or neurogenic causes.[3]

The goals of treatment of PAD are to reduce CVD morbidity and mortality, prevent disease progression, and improve quality of life by alleviating symptoms.[3] The clinical management of patients with PAD involves the aggressive modification of CVD risk factors by lifestyle changes and pharmacologic intervention.[3] Smoking cessation, adequate management of HTN, diabetes, and dyslipidemia, as well as administration of antiplatelet agents reduce CVD morbidity and mortality.[3] Regarding dyslipidemia, the Heart Protection Study showed that treatment with statins (namely simvastatin) significantly reduces the risk for CVD events in patients with PAD.[8] Statins also appear to improve renal function in patients with PAD.[9]

Regarding the management of intermittent claudication, supervised exercise training and the administration of cilostazol, pentoxifylline, or other vasodilators may improve pain-free and maximal walking distance.[3] In symptomatic patients who are unresponsive to the above therapies, revascularization with endovascular procedures or surgical intervention is recommended to relieve symptoms and improve quality of life.[3]

According to the American College of Cardiology/American Heart Association (ACC/AHA) guidelines, the goal of antihypertensive treatment is to achieve BP levels below 140/90 mm Hg in patients without diabetes or below 130/80 mm Hg in patients with diabetes or CKD to reduce CVD morbidity and mortality.[3] The five major classes of antihypertensive drugs (diuretics, beta-blockers, CCBs, ACE inhibitors, and ARBs) are all effective for the management of HTN in patients with PAD.[3]

A meta-analysis of randomized controlled trials using beta-blockers in PAD showed no significant worsening of intermittent claudication or walking distance.[3] The newer beta-blockers, such as nebivolol or carvedilol, may offer additional advantages due to the nitric oxide release-mediated vasodilatation or to their antioxidant properties.[3] A substudy of the Heart Outcomes Prevention Evaluation (HOPE) trial showed that the ACE inhibitor ramipril reduced the risk of MI, stroke, or CVD death by 25% in patients with symptomatic PAD compared with placebo.[10] The use of ACE inhibitors in patients with asymptomatic PAD is less well established.[3] In a substudy of the Valsartan Antihypertensive Long-term Use Evaluation (VALUE) trial, there was no significant difference in CVD events in PAD patients treated either with the ARB valsartan or the CCB amlodipine.[11]

Two studies showed that intensive BP lowering compared with usual management of HTN reduces high CVD risk in PAD patients—in the International Verapamil-Trandolapril (INVEST) study, the ACE inhibitor trandolapril and the diuretic hydrochlorothiazide were added to prior treatment based on the CCB verapamil or the beta-blocker atenolol, and the Appropriate Blood Pressure Control in Diabetes (ABCD) study compared the CCB nisoldipine with the ACE inhibitor enalapril.[12,13]

Summary

PAD is not a localized disease but represents a manifestation of atherosclerosis in the peripheral arterial bed. Therefore, PAD indicates an increased risk for CHD, MI, stroke, and CVD death. Early diagnosis through ABI measurement, even in patients without typical symptoms, and prompt management with aggressive lifestyle modification, appropriate use of combination drug therapy, and (when needed) invasive treatment can greatly reduce CVD morbidity and mortality in this high-risk population.

References

1. Hirsch AT, Criqui MH, Treat-Jacobson D, et al. Peripheral arterial disease detection, awareness, and treatment in primary care. *JAMA* 2001;286:1317–1324.

2. Missouris CG, Buckenham T, Cappuccio FP, MacGregor GA. Renal artery stenosis: a common and important problem in patients with peripheral vascular disease. *Am J Med* 1994;96:10–14.

3. ACC/AHA 2005 guidelines for the management of patients with peripheral arterial disease (lower extremity, renal, mesenteric, and abdominal aortic): executive summary a collaborative report from the American Association for Vascular Surgery/Society for Vascular Surgery, Society for Cardiovascular Angiography and Interventions, Society for Vascular Medicine and Biology, Society of Interventional Radiology, and the ACC/AHA Task Force on Practice Guidelines (Writing Committee to Develop Guidelines for the Management of Patients

With Peripheral Arterial Disease) endorsed by the American Association of Cardiovascular and Pulmonary Rehabilitation; National Heart, Lung, and Blood Institute; Society for Vascular Nursing; TransAtlantic Inter-Society Consensus; and Vascular Disease Foundation. *J Am Coll Cardiol* 2006;47:1239–1312.

4. Tziomalos K, Athyros VG, Karagiannis A, Mikhailidis DP. The role of ankle brachial index and carotid intima-media thickness in vascular risk stratification. *Curr Opin Cardiol* 2010;25:394–398.

5. Karagiannis A, Balaska K, Tziomalos K, et al. Lack of an association between angiotensin converting enzyme gene polymorphism and peripheral arterial occlusive disease. *Vasc Med* 2004;9:189–192.

6. Steg PG, Bhatt DL, Wilson PW, et al. One-year cardiovascular event rates in outpatients with atherothrombosis. *JAMA* 2007;297:1197–1206.

7. Ohman EM, Bhatt DL, Steg PG, et al. The Reduction of Atherothrombosis for Continued Health (REACH) Registry: an international, prospective, observational investigation in subjects at risk for atherothrombotic events-study design. *Am Heart J* 2006;151:786.e1–10.

8. Heart Protection Study Collaborative Group. Randomized trial of the effects of cholesterol-lowering with simvastatin on peripheral vascular and other major vascular outcomes in 20,536 people with peripheral arterial disease and other high-risk conditions. *J Vasc Surg* 2007;45:645–654.

9. Youssef F, Gupta P, Seifalian AM, Myint F, Mikhailidis DP, Hamilton G. The effect of short-term treatment with simvastatin on renal function in patients with peripheral arterial disease. *Angiology* 2004;55:53–62.

10. Ostergren J, Sleight P, Dagenais G, et al. Impact of ramipril in patients with evidence of clinical or subclinical peripheral arterial disease. *Eur Heart J* 2004;25:17–24.

11. Zanchetti A, Julius S, Kjeldsen S, et al. Outcomes in subgroups of hypertensive patients treated with regimens based on valsartan and amlodipine: An analysis of findings from the VALUE trial. *J Hypertens* 2006;24:2163–2168.

12. Pepine CJ, Kowey PR, Kupfer S, et al. Predictors of adverse outcome among patients with hypertension and coronary artery disease. *J Am Coll Cardiol* 2006;47:547–551.

13. Mehler PS, Coll JR, Estacio R, Esler A, Schrier RW, Hiatt WR. Intensive blood pressure control reduces the risk of cardiovascular events in patients with peripheral arterial disease and type 2 diabetes. *Circulation* 2003;107:753–756.

Improving Hypertension Control

a. Adherence to Regimens

David Martins, MD, MS, Nosratola D. Vaziri, MD, and Keith Norris, MD

A 55-year-old woman with a 6-year history of HTN and a 4-year history of type 2 diabetes presents for follow-up of BP. Her BMI has been high (33 kg/m²) and BP control has been inconsistent. Her medications include ramipril 10 mg daily and hydrochlorothiazide 25 mg daily for HTN. Her BP is now 156/98 mm Hg. You inquire about her adherence to her medication regimen and she admits to occasional lapses in taking her pills. You probe further into other potential issues, such as the cost of medications and side effects. She states her insurance does cover the cost, although there is a modest co-pay that is constantly increasing. There do not seem to be any significant side effects, but you remind her to bring any possible side effects to your attention so that you can modify her medications if necessary. You reinforce the importance of adherence to medications and diet, and she feels reinvigorated and vows to be more compliant. Two weeks later, her BP is 144/86 mm Hg. You remark on the significant improvement in her BP but that because of coexisting diabetes her BP goal is not the usual less than 140/90 mm Hg but a lower goal of less than 130/80 mm Hg. Again you reinforce the importance of adherence to medications and diet, and prescribe extended-release diltiazem 180 mg daily to help reach the goal BP. Two weeks later, her BP is 126/78 mm Hg and she remains asymptomatic. You commend her on doing an excellent job and note that over time, with aggressive lifestyle modifications and weight loss, you may be able to reduce her medications.

High BP or HTN, defined as untreated SBP of 140 mm Hg or higher or DBP of 90 mm Hg or higher, taking antihypertensive medicine, or being told at least twice by a health professional, affects one in three U.S. adults, or over 74 million Americans.[1] HTN is the most common diagnosis for ambulatory medical illness, and one of the major risk factors for developing CV and related diseases, the leading cause of death in the nation. Data from the Framingham Heart Study indicate that HTN is associated with shorter overall life expectancy. At age 50, total life expectancy is 5 shorter in those with HTN than in those with normal BP. The estimated direct and indirect cost of HTN for 2009 was $73.4 billion, while the cost of associated CVD was nearly $500 billion. Despite major advances in HTN therapies, from 1996 to 2006, the age-adjusted death rate from HTN increased 20% and the actual number of deaths rose 48%.[1] Data from NHANES 2003–2006 showed that of those with HTN age 20 and older, 78% were aware of their condition and 68% were under current treatment, while only 44% had their BP under control.[1] Unfortunately, that means over 50% did not have their BP controlled.

Several factors can contribute to difficulty in achieving optimal BP control, and one of the most important factors is adherence to therapeutic regimens and lifestyle modifications.

Adherence and Health Care Costs

Broadly, lack of adherence can come in many forms, such as receiving a prescription but not filling it, increasing or decreasing the frequency of doses, missing office visits, and others (Table 7a.1). Lack of adherence to antihypertensive medications and CV lifestyle recommendations causes not only personal hardship due to accelerated morbidity and mortality, but also societal hardship from increased health care costs. Pittman et al. performed a retrospective analysis of adherence using the medication possession ratio and its association with health care costs and CV-related hospitalizations and emergency department visits using a national pharmacy benefits database of over 625,000 patients with a diagnosis of HTN. They identified 62,388 persons (10%) with less than 60% adherence (low), 96,226 (15%) with 60% to 79% adherence (moderate), and 467,006 patients (75%) with 80% or higher adherence (high). Patients with high adherence were more likely to be older and male, to have higher chronic disease scores and lower antihypertensive medication co-payments, and to fill a greater percentage of prescriptions by mail order. Patients with high adherence had significantly lower age- and sex-adjusted odds of CV-related hospitalizations, emergency department visits, and adjusted health care costs than the moderate and low adherence groups.[2] Similar findings were reported in a cohort of 59,647 Canadian patients between 45 and 85 years of age with essential HTN and no evidence for symptomatic CV disease.[3]

Table 7a.1 Type of Non-adherence
Receiving a prescription but not filling it
Running out of medicine
Not having BP medicine available when it is time to take a dose
Taking an incorrect dose
Taking medication at the wrong times
Increasing or decreasing the frequency of doses
Stopping the treatment too soon
Delay in seeking health care
Non-participation in clinic visits
Failure to follow doctor's instructions
"Drug holidays": patient stops therapy for a while and then restarts the therapy
"White coat adherence": patients are adherent around the time of clinic appointments
(Source: Jin J, Sklar GE, Min Sen Oh V, Chuen Li S. Factors affecting therapeutic compliance: A review from the patient's perspective. *Ther Clin Risk Manag* 2008;4(1):269–286.)

Adherence and Clinical Outcomes

Adherence to BP control can be categorized into five major groups of key risk factors: patient-centered, therapy-related, health care system, social and economic, and disease-related (Table 7a.2).[4–6] Several of these risk factors for adherence to BP control are behavioral and modifiable. The identification and communication of the risk attributable to behaviors (e.g., dietary indiscretion,

Table 7a.2 Categories of Factors that Influence Adherence	
Patient-centered factors	Demographic factors: age, ethnicity, gender, education, marital status
	Psychosocial factors: beliefs, motivation, attitude
	Patient–prescriber relationship: trust, confidence, respect
	Health literacy
	Patient knowledge
	Physical difficulties
	Tobacco, smoking, alcohol intake, or substance abuse
	Forgetfulness: disease- or medication-related
	History of good compliance: highly motivated, self-efficacious
Therapy-related factors	Route of administration
	Treatment complexity
	Duration of the treatment period
	Medication side effects
	Degree of behavioral change required
	Change in one's daily routine
	Taste of the medication
	Requirements for drug storage
Health care system factors	Lack of accessibility
	Long waiting time
	Difficulty in getting prescriptions filled
	Unhappy clinic visits
	Trust or distrust of the provider or the health system
Social and economic factors	Inability to take time off work
	Inability to take time from child care or elder care
	Cost of therapy
	Adequacy of community assets to support healthy CV lifestyle
	Social support
Disease factors	Disease symptoms or lack of symptoms
	Severity of the disease: impact on memory, impact on healthy CV lifestyle
	Depression: disease-related, medication-related, other

(Source: Jin J, Sklar GE, Min Sen Oh V, Chuen Li S. Factors affecting therapeutic compliance: A review from the patient's perspective. *Ther Clin Risk Manag* 2008;4(1):269–286.)

physical inactivity, excessive alcohol intake, and smoking), particularly within the context of established CVD burden, should engage and encourage the patient to be proactive in risk-reduction strategies (Table 7a.3).[7] However, effective communication necessitates compassion and concern by the health

Table 7a.3 Select Considerations and Strategies for Improving Adherence	
Cultural	
Overweight/obese (BMI >25/30 kg/m²) Negotiation for an intermediate goal is often needed.	In some communities there is cultural concern that a thin body habitus is associated with poor health.
High dietary intake of sodium and fat Chance to recognize cultural values and negotiate an intermediate goal while gaining trust and respect	Cultural food preparation and/or conditioned tasting continued from eras when high salt and fat content were needed for preservation and/or palatability of suboptimal food sources
Low dietary calcium intake Inquire about food intolerances.	Low milk and dairy intake may be due to lactose intolerance.
Inactivity for women May not be immediately obvious to patient as a barrier	Relatively high cost of hairstyling and hair maintenance may contribute to avoidance of exercising or limiting swimming or exercising to the point of increased heart rate and sweating.
Traditional Medical	

Low adherence to prescribed treatment plan
 	
Be proactive in assessing cost of therapy and side effects. Many patients will be unwilling to volunteer side effects and too proud to volunteer cost issues.
	• Assess for medication side effects (e.g., impotence, cough, nightmares).
	• Ask patients if they have insurance.
	  • If yes, does their insurance cover the prescribed medication? Is the co-pay affordable?
	  • If no, can they afford the prescribed medications, or might they prefer a lower-cost medication in a different class (e.g., generic diuretic or beta-blocker)?

Missed office appointments Be flexible and proactive in arranging visits that are more likely to be adhered to.	• Transportation difficulties: Patients may not have a car, and many cities have poor mass transportation systems. • Competing priorities such as child/grandchild care, elder care (often related to extended family home structure; child care and elder care facilities are often geographically disconnected from health centers) • Limited ability to leave work to attend health care appointments in many job settings
(Source: Norris KC, Tareen N, Martins D, Vaziri N. Implications of ethnicity for the treatment of hypertensive kidney disease, with an emphasis on African Americans. *Nat Clin Pract Nephrol* 2008;4(10):538–549.)	

care provider to engender a sense of trust. Dietary strategies for BP control and overall CV risk reduction should recognize and reiterate the therapeutic impact of therapeutic lifestyle changes.[8] The DASH study achieved 5- to 10-mm Hg reductions in SBP among participants on the study diet versus a control diet and was effective for African-Americans, a cohort for whom it is traditionally more difficult to achieve BP control. While this was an extremely controlled environment, with prepared food provided to study participants, a diet similar to that used in the DASH study should yield improved BPs for most patients with HTN.

Other factors are more difficult to address but equally important to assess and integrate into a comprehensive care plan, such as insurance status. Lack of insurance is associated with lower rates of BP control among treated but not among untreated persons with HTN, likely related to differences in appropriate treatment intensification or adherence rather than differences in rates of treatment initiation.[9] Assessing a patient's insurance medication coverage and adjusting therapy accordingly can play an important role in enhancing adherence. Other health care system factors are highlighted in Table 7a.2. Adherence interventions have yielded mixed results. Pladevall et al. randomized 877 patients with uncontrolled HTN to a multifactorial intervention group where physicians counted patients' pills, designated a family member to support adherence behavior, and provided educational information to patients or usual care. Intervention patients were almost half as likely to have uncontrolled SBP and nearly twice as likely to be adherent at 6 months. However, after 5 years of follow-up there was no difference in long-term CV events.[10] Further studies are needed to assess the impact of adherence approaches on long-term outcomes.

As noted in the vignette, reinforcing adherence to medications and diet is paramount for improving BP control. A comprehensive approach to CV risk reduction in addition to achieving optimal BP should include lifestyle modifications, glycemic and lipid control, low-dose acetylsalicylic acid (unless contraindicated), and smoking cessation, if applicable. Many people with type 2 diabetes and HTN will need three or more drugs to control HTN to the target BP of below 130/80. In addition, the administration of multiple medications often allows the use of lower doses that can minimize side effects while addressing several neurohormonal systems and/or potential risk factors that may contribute to complications. To provide vascular protection therapy directed at inhibition of the rennin-angiotensin system with ACE inhibitors or ARBs is a common initial therapy as it helps to prevent diabetes complications. Low-dose diuretics are synergistic with ACE inhibitors and ARBs in lowering BP and are frequently needed to achieve target BP goals. A long-acting CCB, particularly a non-dihydropyridine CCB (e.g., diltiazem, verapamil) should be considered for proteinuric hypertensive patients such as those with diabetic nephropathy, since they have been shown to reduce urinary albumin excretion. Additional options include cardioselective beta-blockers and alpha-adrenergic blockers or others, depending on coexisting medical conditions.

Conclusion

HTN treatment should be driven, in part, not only by the prevalence of coexisting CV risk factors but also the prevailing socioeconomic context, integrated into a effective real-world treatment plan for an individual patient. In addition to selecting the most appropriate pharmacologic therapies, achieving optimal outcomes necessitates an appropriate sensitivity to and an understanding of the unique sociocultural and economic aspects to maximize access to care, adherence to treatment, and scheduled follow-up. For optimal HTN control, the clinician must take into account demographic and sociocultural factors such as race/ethnicity, gender, age, employment, income, leisure time availability, poverty, family support, education, medical insurance status, and others that may act as barriers to adherence. Such approaches will ultimately assist in overcoming many of the barriers to HTN control and improve CV outcomes. Effective long-term interventions are needed not only to improve adherence and BP control, but also to reduce health care costs and improve CV outcomes.

Acknowledgments

Supported in part by NIH Grants U54 RR026138 and P20 MD00182.

References

1. American Heart Association. *Heart Disease and Stroke Statistics—2010 Update.* Dallas: AHA, 2010.

2. Pittman DG, Tao Z, Chen W, Stettin GD. Antihypertensive medication adherence and subsequent healthcare utilization and costs. *Am J Manag Care* 2010;16(8):568–576.

3. Dragomir A, Côté R, Roy L, Blais L, Lalonde L, Bérard A, Perreault S. Impact of adherence to antihypertensive agents on clinical outcomes and hospitalization costs. *Med Care* 2010;48(5):418–425.

4. Martin MY, Kohler C, Kim YI, Kratt P, Schoenberger YM, Litaker MS, Prayor-Patterson HM, Clarke SJ, Andrews S, Pisu M. Original paper: taking less than prescribed: medication nonadherence and provider-patient relationships in lower-income, rural minority adults with hypertension. *J Clin Hypertens* 2010;12(9):706–713.

5. Aggarwal B, Mosca L. Lifestyle and psychosocial risk factors predict non-adherence to medication. *Ann Behav Med* 2010;40(2):228–233.

6. Jin J, Sklar GE, Min Sen Oh V, Chuen Li S. Factors affecting therapeutic compliance: A review from the patient's perspective. *Ther Clin Risk Manag* 2008;4(1):269–286.

7. Norris KC, Tareen N, Martins D, Vaziri N. Implications of ethnicity for the treatment of hypertensive kidney disease, with an emphasis on African Americans. *Nat Clin Pract Nephrol* 2008;4(10):538–549.

8. Chobanian AV, Bakris GL, Black HR, Cushman WC, Green LA, Izzo JL Jr, Jones DW, Materson BJ, Oparil S, Wright JT Jr, Roccella EJ; Joint National Committee on Prevention, Detection, Evaluation, and Treatment of High Blood Pressure, National Heart, Lung, and Blood Institute, National High Blood Pressure Education Program Coordinating Committee. Seventh report of the Joint National Committee on Prevention, Detection, Evaluation and Treatment of High Blood Pressure. *Hypertension.* 2003;42:1206–1252.

9. Duru OK, Vargas RB, Kermah D, Pan D, Norris KC. Health insurance status and hypertension monitoring and control in the United States. *Am J Hypertens* 2007;20(4):348–353.

10. Pladevall M, Brotons C, Gabriel R, Arnau A, Suarez C, de la Figuera M, Marquez E, Coca A, Sobrino J, Divine G, Heisler M, Williams LK; Writing Committee on behalf of the COM99 Study Group. Multicenter cluster-randomized trial of a multifactorial intervention to improve antihypertensive medication adherence and blood pressure control among patients at high cardiovascular risk (the COM99 study). *Circulation* 2010;122(12):1183–1191.

b. Resistant Hypertension

Domenic A. Sica, MD

This patient is a 62-year-old black man with a longstanding history of HTN that has become increasingly difficult to control over the past several months. He takes his BP at home routinely and it rarely varies from the values obtained in his physician's office. He offers few symptoms other than daytime fatigue, dry mouth, and some shortness of breath with exercise. He denies anxiety, depression, and panic attacks and does not snore or awaken gasping for air. He denies use of any over-the-counter medications, high-dose vitamins, or herbal products. He has a normal physical examination other than trace peripheral edema. His BP is 180/105 mm Hg in the right arm and he is not orthostatic. His heart rate is 48 bpm and he weighs 230 pounds, with a body mass index of 34 kg/m^2. He currently is on a six-drug regimen, including maximum doses of atenolol (100 mg twice daily), hydrochlorothiazide (50 mg/day), lisinopril (40 mg/day), amlodipine (10 mg twice daily), candesartan (32 mg/day), and clonidine (0.2 mg three times daily). His initial screening laboratory studies include serum potassium 3.4 mmol/L, serum sodium 137 mmol/L, serum creatinine 1.04 mg/dL, serum calcium 9.8 mg/dL, and serum hemoglobin 16 g/dL.

Resistant HTN is an everyday clinical problem dealt with by both primary care clinicians and specialists alike. While the exact prevalence of resistant HTN is debated, clinical trials suggest that it occurs in as many as 30% of study participants. Central obesity and older age are consistent risk factors for resistant HTN, and as the population ages and gains weight it can be expected that its prevalence will rise further. Certain subsets of patients are also more at risk for the development of resistant HTN, including those with diabetes, sleep apnea, chronic kidney disease (CKD), LV hypertrophy, mood disorders, an excessively high sodium (Na$^+$) intake, and undue sympathetic nervous system (SNS) activation.[1,2]

Definition

Resistant HTN is defined in order to categorize patients who are at high risk of having reversible causes of HTN and/or patients who, because of persistently high BP levels, may benefit from special diagnostic and therapeutic approaches; however, the definition of the term "resistant HTN" is not universally agreed upon, and its varying definitions can be the source of some confusion. Resistant HTN is best defined as a BP reading that remains above goal despite the concurrent use of three antihypertensive agents of different classes given at optimal dose amounts, with one of these three agents if at all possible being a diuretic.

Although arbitrary in regard to the number of medications required, as defined, resistant HTN includes patients whose BP is at goal with more than three medications; thus, patients whose BP is at goal but only with the use of four or more medications would be defined as having resistant HTN.[1]

Evaluation and Management

The evaluation of patients with resistant HTN should be directed toward verifying true resistance to treatment; recognizing factors causal for treatment resistance, including secondary causes of HTN; and documenting target-organ damage. Management of resistant HTN begins with a thorough evaluation of the patient to both verify the diagnosis and to rule out pseudo-resistance (Table 7b.1). Improper BP measurement technique, white coat effect, and poor patient adherence to lifestyle and/or prescribed antihypertensive medications are major pseudo-resistance considerations. For the patient presented at the beginning of the chapter, pseudo-resistance was not a concern in that his BP was measured with an appropriately sized cuff, he had nothing to suggest white coat HTN (comparable office and home BP readings), and he was meticulous in his medication taking, as confirmed by his wife. Clinical inertia also was not an issue in that his physician had systematically titrated up his antihypertensive medications and sequentially added different medication classes such that he was now on a six-drug regimen.[3]

Education and reinforcement of health care practices that lower BP, such as dietary Na^+ restriction, cutting back on alcohol intake, and weight loss if obese, are essential in treating resistant HTN. Excessive dietary Na^+ is rife in patients with resistant HTN, and in such patients obtaining a random 24-hour urine for Na^+ excretion can prove quite useful in crafting future dietary recommendations. Heavy alcohol intake is associated with both an increased risk of HTN as well as the development of treatment-resistant HTN. The threshold above

Table 7b.1 Causes of Pseudo-resistance in the Patient with Resistant HTN
Poor BP measurement technique
Poorly compressible arm arteries in patients with heavily calcified blood vessels
White coat phenomenon
Patient non-adherence
Medication cost
Poorly coordinated dosing schedules
Medication side effects
Memory or psychiatric issues
Cultural acceptance of medications
Poorly delivered patient instructions
Excessive dose titration and use of medications that are poorly complementary
Physician inertia

which alcohol became deleterious for HTN risk is patient-specific but in some studies has been shown to emerge at more than four drinks a day in women and as little as more than one drink/day in men.[4] In addition, binge drinking can have a prominent yet rapidly reversible effect on BP, which presents as resistant HTN intermingled with periods of well-controlled HTN. In our patient his weight had been stable, he abstained from drinking, and he was vigilant with restricting his Na^+ intake; thus, these health care practices did not need to be further addressed relative to his resistant HTN.

A number of medication classes and over-the-counter products can increase BP and as such become factors in treatment resistance (Table 7b.2). The effects of these agents can be highly individualized, with most manifesting little or no effect, while other individuals may experience severe and unremitting elevations in BP. A cause-and-effect relationship between these compounds and HTN often goes unrecognized by health care providers unless questioning is quite specific. Even with the most precise questioning the contribution of over-the-counter medications to a particular pattern of HTN may go undetected in that a number of weight-loss products have now been found to be tainted with compounds such as sibutramine.

Although recommendations for the pharmacologic treatment of resistant HTN remain largely empiric, there are several components of the treatment plan that need to be systematically addressed even as the search for secondary causes of HTN is undertaken (Table 7b.3).[5]

Upward dose titration of medications often occurs with the best of intentions. However, most antihypertensive medications have a flat to shallow dose–response curve; thus, after the first dose doubling, further dose increases

Table 7b.2 Medications that Can Interfere with BP Control
Alcohol
Oral contraceptives
Corticosteroids
Nonsteroidal anti-inflammatory drugs
Cyclooxygenase-2 inhibitors
Sympathomimetic amines
Decongestants
Weight-loss–promoting agents
Cocaine
Stimulants
Methylphenidate
Dexmethylphenidate
Dextroamphetamine
Cyclosporine
Erythropoiesis-stimulating agents
Natural licorice
Tainted over-the-counter weight-loss products
Sibutramine

Table 7b.3 Elements of the Treatment Plan for Resistant HTN
Avoid excessive dose titration for drugs with a flat dose–response for BP reduction.
Consider split dosing of medications.
Use home BP measurement to assist in medication timing.
Establish heart rate control (<70 bpm).
Improve sleep quality.
Recognize and treat anxiety/depression.
Optimize diuretic therapy to keep the patient euvolemic.
Identify rebound HTN in patients treated with central-alpha agonists.

generally are of little use. This is not the case for side effects, however, which are strongly dose-dependent. The fatigue our patient is experiencing is most likely due to the inordinately high dose of atenolol being used. Many medications are labeled as once-daily medications, but in the patient with resistant HTN their duration of action is in many instances substantially less. Home BP monitoring can determine how long a medication or grouping of medications truly effect a reduction in BP. Stated otherwise, in the patient with resistant HTN many once-daily medications lose their effect well before the end of a 24-hour dose interval and as such require a supplemental dose be given. The use of a second medication dose, typically given in the evening hours, will preferentially reduce BP when asleep with its attendant benefits.[6] Careful attention to the sleep–wake cycle can sometimes have a significant effect on BP in that the patient with resistant HTN and obstructive sleep apnea has shorter overall and REM sleep times, independent of the level of sleep apnea.[7]

Heart rate control is an additional consideration in the treatment of resistant HTN. Heart rate can be elevated as a primary factor in some forms of resistant HTN as well as being a secondary response to nonspecific vasodilators, such as hydralazine or minoxidil.[8] In most cases, careful control of heart rate is a prerequisite to achieving BP control in the patient with resistant HTN. It is recognized that anxiety and panic are characterized by a range of physiologic symptoms such as tachycardia, sweating, flushing, and shaking; what is less appreciated is that the activation of the SNS that marks these mood disorders can prove the basis for a patient having resistant HTN.[9]

Patients with resistant HTN frequently have inappropriate volume expansion contributing to their treatment resistance such that a diuretic is essential if BP control is to be optimized. In most patients, use of a long-acting thiazide-type diuretic will accomplish this goal;[10] however, in patients with underlying CKD, loop diuretics may be necessary for effective volume and BP control. Furosemide is a relatively short-acting loop diuretic and typically requires at least twice-daily dosing; alternatively, loop diuretics with a longer duration of action, such as torsemide, are available and can be given on a once-daily basis.[11]

In our patient, several changes were made to his regimen: (1) reducing the atenolol dose from 100 mg twice daily to 50 mg once daily (flat dose–response curve above 50 mg/day); (2) discontinuing the candesartan (redundant effect on BP when given with an ACE inhibitor); (3) discontinuing the clonidine 0.2 mg three times daily and substituting a transdermal clonidine patch #2 (to lessen the side effects seen with oral clonidine); and (4) discontinuing the hydrochlorothiazide 50 mg/day and substituting chlorthalidone 25 mg once daily (to provide a more long-acting thiazide-type diuretic). With these changes his BP fell into the 155–160/90–95 mm Hg range and he felt less fatigued. His ongoing workup showed him to have a plasma aldosterone value of 20 ng/dL (normal range 1 to 16 ng/dL) and a plasma renin activity value of less than 0.15 ng/mL/hr (normal range 0.5 to 2.5 ng/mL/hr). He was then started on spironolactone 25 mg twice daily, and within 2 weeks his BP dropped to the 125–130/75–80 mm Hg range. Completion of his workup for aldosteronism showed him to have elevated urine aldosterone excretion and a 2-cm left adrenal adenoma on adrenal imaging.

Conclusions

Resistant HTN is a multicomponent disorder with numerous contributing factors; however, if the patient with resistant HTN is systematically approached, goal BP can often be reached. Secondary causes of HTN, such as aldosteronism, should be sought in the patient with resistant HTN since the drop in BP can be quite dramatic with specific treatment of a secondary cause.

References

1. Calhoun DA, Jones D, Textor S, et al. Resistant hypertension: diagnosis, evaluation, and treatment. A scientific statement from the American Heart Association Professional Education Committee of the Council for High Blood Pressure Research. *Hypertension* 2008;51:1403–1419.

2. Sarafidis PA, Bakris GL. Resistant hypertension: an overview of evaluation and treatment. *J Am Coll Cardiol* 2008;52:1749–1757.

3. Okonofua EC, Simpson KN, Jesri A, et al. Therapeutic inertia is an impediment to achieving the Healthy People 2010 blood pressure control goals. *Hypertension* 2006;47:345–351.

4. Sesso HD, Cook NR, Buring JE, et al. Alcohol consumption and the risk of hypertension in women and men. *Hypertension* 2008;51:1080–1087.

5. Parthasarathy HK, Alhashmi K, McMahon AD, et al. Does the ratio of serum aldosterone to plasma renin activity predict the efficacy of diuretics in hypertension? Results of RENALDO. *J Hypertens* 2010;28:170–177.

6. Smolensky MH, Hermida RC, Ayala DE, et al. Administration-time-dependent effects of blood pressure-lowering medications: basis for the chronotherapy of hypertension. *Blood Press Monit* 2010;15:173–180.

7. Friedman O, Bradley TD, Ruttanaumpawan P, Logan AG. Independent association of drug-resistant hypertension to reduced sleep duration and efficiency. *Am J Hypertens* 2010;23:174–179.

8. Kolloch R, Legler UF, Champion A, et al. Impact of resting heart rate on outcomes in hypertensive patients with coronary artery disease: findings from the International VErapamil-SR/trandolapril STudy (INVEST). *Eur Heart J* 2008;29:1327–1334.

9. Davies SJ, Esler M, Nutt DJ. Anxiety: bridging the heart/mind divide. *J Psychopharmacol* 2010;24:633–638.

10. Sica DA. Chlorthalidone: has it always been the best thiazide-type diuretic? *Hypertension* 2006;47:321–322.

11. Sica D, Carl D. Pathologic basis and treatment considerations in chronic kidney disease-related hypertension. *Sem Nephrol* 2005;25:246–251.

Chapter 8

Public Health Challenges and Community Programs

Paula T. Einhorn, MD, MS

HTN is a modifiable risk factor for stroke, heart failure, MI, and renal failure. Defined as SBP greater than 140 mm Hg and/or DBP greater than 90 mm Hg or on treatment, it affects about a third of the United States population (over 70 million) and about a billion individuals worldwide, and thus presents a formidable public health challenge for both the United States and the global community.[1–3]

HTN Is Treatable

Systematic treatment of HTN (compared with a placebo or usual care) has been shown to reduce stroke by about 40%; heart failure, especially with preserved LV ejection fraction, by up to 65%; MI by about 20%; and premature mortality by about 20%.[4] Diagnosing HTN does not require invasive testing and is very simple and inexpensive. However, the disease is asymptomatic, and thus there is an important role for the community to identify hypertensive individuals, and enable and motivate them to seek medical advice and then stay on treatment.

HTN Is Preventable

In industrialized countries, the prevalence of HTN increases dramatically with age. However, some persons, including those whose diets consist mostly of vegetable products and those whose sodium intake is low, have virtually no increase in HTN with age.[3] Prevention or delay of the onset of HTN can prevent or at least postpone the long-term clinical sequelae of elevated BP and, thus, prevent premature mortality and disability.

Prevention of HTN begins in childhood and continues through adulthood.[5] Decades of NHLBI-sponsored research have developed dietary approaches to stop HTN (DASH diet) and documented long-term benefits of dietary sodium reduction.[3] In addition, a recent publication showed that for overweight or obese individuals with above-normal BP (SBP 130 to 159 or DBP 85 to 99 mm Hg), the addition of exercise and weight loss to the DASH diet resulted in an even larger BP reduction than the DASH diet alone.[6] Given the documented value of lifestyle changes, including those leading to achieving or maintaining healthy body weight, community involvement is of paramount importance for prevention of HTN. While individuals at higher risk, such as adults and children with pre-HTN and those with diabetes and/or a history of CVD, may require individual counseling, the rest of the population at risk— which is virtually everyone—needs a community with an environment and culture conducive to maintenance of normal BP.

The Community

Let us define this community. HTN is a global problem affecting both developed and underdeveloped countries. The disease is both preventable and treatable; thus, the community includes both lay individuals and health professionals, and organizational structures associated with these individuals. It's a major public health problem and thus requires involvement of public health organizations and governmental structures.

Disparities

HTN affects individuals of all racial and ethnic backgrounds, men and women, of all socioeconomic strata. However, differences in the prevalence, treatment, and control of HTN, and the age of onset, provide justification for targeted approaches. Black individuals have been long recognized to have the earliest onset and the highest prevalence of HTN, which underscores the importance of prevention.[1,2,4,5,7] But after decades of community involvement (e.g., faith-based organizations, barber and beauty shops) guided by results of rigorous research, black individuals have the highest levels of awareness and treatment of HTN. Awareness and treatment rates are the lowest among Hispanics, especially those aged less than 60, where the potential for preventing long-term clinical outcomes is the greatest. The rate of BP control among treated hypertensive individuals has greatly improved over the past two decades, especially among non-Hispanic white men aged less than 60. The disparity in this area continues for black individuals and women, despite clear evidence of long-term benefits of treatment. Clinical trial evidence for BP control in the very elderly has only recently become available.[1,2,4,7]

What Has Been Accomplished and What Needs To Be Done

The past four decades have witnessed remarkable improvements in HTN awareness, treatment, and control. In a recent publication, Egan et al. describe these accomplishments and also recognize the persistence of the demographic disparities.[7] To increase BP control in all groups, they recommend broad-based efforts to further improve awareness, treatment, and proportions of patients treated and controlled. They also note the importance of complementary programs to (1) raise awareness and treatment among 18- to 39-year-old persons, Hispanics, and men, and (2) increase the proportion of patients treated and controlled among persons 60 years or older, blacks, and women for improving HTN control and reducing disparities.

The National High Blood Pressure Education Program (NHBPEP), a cooperative effort among professional and voluntary health agencies, state health departments, and many community groups, was established in 1972 and coordinated by NHLBI (http://hp2010.nhlbihin.net/nhbpep.htm). With the overarching goal to reduce death and disability related to HTN through programs of professional, patient, and public education, the NHBPEP has made meaningful contributions not only towards the achievement of the Healthy People 2010 Objectives for the Nation but also to the 64% decline in the age-adjusted CV mortality rates that has occurred since 1963.

Recently, the Institute of Medicine (IOM) panel has declared HTN a "neglected disease" that costs the U.S. health care system $73 billion per year. The panel recognized that attacking HTN from the aspect of public policy and systems is realistic and practical.[8] This important recognition gives new impetus to the decades of efforts to reduce the burden and consequences of HTN.

Individuals at Risk for HTN

As noted by the IOM chair, Dr. David Fleming of the Public Health Department of Seattle and King County, Washington, individuals who live long enough are almost guaranteed to develop HTN.[8] Thus, increased longevity inevitably leads to an increase in the prevalence of HTN, and so does increased survival of individuals with HTN and with conditions predisposing to the development of HTN, such as chronic kidney disease, coronary heart disease, and diabetes. The only way to reduce the prevalence of HTN is to prevent or delay its onset. Given that virtually everyone is at risk, this can be accomplished only by targeting the entire population—that is, by using public health approaches involving all communities yet tailored to the specific needs of individual communities.

Obesity is an established risk factor for HTN. NHLBI and NIDDK lead the NIH efforts to combat the epidemic of obesity through research and community programs. Recently completed NHLBI-sponsored studies, including those in schools and worksites, will inform these efforts, as will the results of ongoing studies targeting adolescents and young adults and assessing interventions to reduce obesity in ambulatory clinical settings. A $49.5 million Childhood Obesity Prevention and Treatment Research (COPTR) program will support randomized clinical trials to prevent and treat obesity in children. A large investment has also been made in evaluation of community programs to reduce childhood obesity rates (http://public.nhlbi.nih.gov/newsroom/home/GetPressRelease.aspx?id=2725).

These programs will undoubtedly make a substantial contribution to HTN prevention. However, not all individuals with HTN are obese, and the recent rise in prevalence of overweight and obesity cannot fully explain the growing prevalence of HTN, especially in women.[1] Thus, population-based approaches need to go beyond targeting obesity and include HTN-specific interventions such as salt intake reduction and DASH diets.[3,5,9] A substantial body of evidence exists to support population-wide efforts to reduce salt intake as means to reduce the burden of HTN and CVD, especially in women and black individuals. Such efforts are already in place in other countries, including Japan, the United Kingdom, Finland, and Portugal. They involve a combination of regulations on salt content in processed foods, labeling of processed and prepared foods, public education, and collaboration with the food industry. In the United States, professional societies, including the American Medical Association, the American Heart Association, and the American Society of Hypertension, have already endorsed population-wide efforts to reduce salt intake, and so did the World Health Organization. The New York City Health Department is setting an example for the national effort to reduce heart attacks and strokes by reducing the amount of salt in packaged and restaurant food through an innovative public–private partnership (http://www.nyc.gov/html/doh/html/cardio/cardio-salt-initiative.shtml). In April 2010, IOM released a report on strategies to reduce sodium intake in the United States. This report, requested by Congress, recommends long-term approaches, including use of regulatory tools in an innovative and unprecedented fashion.[9]

The population-based efforts need to be complemented by (1) continued promotion of the DASH diets (http://www.nhlbi.nih.gov/health/public/heart/hbp/dash/new_dash.pdf) and (2) continued research leading to better understanding of the mechanistic (phenotypic and genetic) underpinnings of BP and target-organ response to diet and exercise for the purpose of further refining and possibly personalizing lifestyle approaches.[3,6]

Individuals with HTN

Those who have already developed HTN need to be under the care of qualified clinicians. Clinical communities alone or in collaboration with lay communities have played an important role in both obtaining the scientific evidence and improving HTN awareness, treatment, and control in the communities. This role will become even greater as researchers and public health practitioners realize the importance of community clinicians and their partners in facilitating and defining the research agenda. Major clinical trials, such as ALLHAT and HDFP, were conducted in the community.[4] By design, they enrolled diverse patient populations and yielded results that influenced clinical practice. In addition to informing guideline development, ALLHAT was the first NIH-funded clinical trial to launch a multi-component program, in collaboration with the NHBPEP, to improve HTN treatment in the community. The program, which disseminated ALLHAT results in the context of the JNC 7 guidelines, used community clinicians as agents of change.[4]

Community plays an important role in identifying individuals with HTN, both within and outside clinical settings. However, the opportunity will be missed if there is no follow-up. There are studies, both completed and ongoing, to inform this process.[2,8] When individuals with HTN become patients with HTN, the primary objective is to achieve BP control for optimal prevention of premature mortality and morbidity. This responsibility rests primarily with clinical researchers and clinicians. Randomized controlled clinical trials have shown that BP control is an achievable goal.[4,8] While questions remain about optimal BP control levels and approaches to combining medications, the evidence for the benefits of BP control to the goal of below 140/90 mm Hg in the majority of patients is very strong. Because HTN is asymptomatic, patients need to understand the chronic nature of the disease and the need to stay on treatment. Fortunately, there is a large body of evidence from rigorously conducted research, including randomized trials, to guide the community programs involving both health practitioners and lay community members.[2,8,10] In addition, studies in progress are evaluating interventions involving all aspects of medical encounters and the environment in which these encounters occur, including interventions to eliminate disparities in HTN control and to incorporate evidence-based lifestyle interventions into routine clinical practice. An important task for the medical community will be to translate these results into clinical practice, while recognizing that no research project can directly apply to every patient and every setting. This is where clinical judgment and common sense come into play. Given the wealth of information already available and soon to be reported, future research needs to build on accomplishments to date and future projects designed through collaborative ventures involving researchers and practitioners.

Conclusions

HTN is an important public health problem because of its global reach and high societal cost, both in dollars and lives lost. In the United States, one third of the adult population has HTN, and virtually everyone else is at risk for the development of HTN. Evidence-based approaches are available for both prevention and treatment of HTN but need to be translated into community practice. Due to the chronic but silent nature of the condition, this will require involvement of a broadly defined community and simultaneous use of population-wide and individual approaches. Community programs need to be evaluated both locally and nationally. Future research needs to be community-responsive and build on past accomplishments.

References

1. Cutler JA, Sorlie PD, Wolz M, Thom T, Fields LE, Roccella EJ. Trends in hypertension prevalence, awareness, treatment, and control rates in United States adults between 1988–1994 and 1999–2004. *Hypertension* 2008;52:818–827.

2. Einhorn PT. National Heart, Lung, and Blood Institute-initiated Program "Interventions to Improve Hypertension Control Rates in African Americans": background and implementation. *Circ Cardiovasc Qual Outcomes* 2009;2(3):236–240.

3. Sacks FM, Campos H. Dietary therapy in hypertension. *N Engl J Med* 2010;362:2102–2112

4. Einhorn PT, Davis BR, Wright JT Jr, Rahman M, Whelton PK, Pressel SL; ALLHAT Cooperative Research Group. ALLHAT: still providing correct answers after 7 years. *Curr Opin Cardiol* 2010;25(4):355–365.

5. Obarzanek E, Wu CO, Cutler JA, Kavey R, Pearson GD, Daniels SR. Prevalence and incidence of hypertension in adolescent girls. *J Pediatr* 2010;157:461–467.

6. Blumenthal JA, Babyak MA, Hinderliter A, et al. Effects of the DASH diet alone and in combination with exercise and weight loss on BP and CV biomarkers in men and women with high BP. The ENCORE study. *Arch Intern Med* 2010;170:126–135.

7. Egan BM, Zhao Y, Neal Axon R, et al. US trends in prevalence, awareness, treatment, and control of hypertension, 1988–2008. *JAMA* 2010;303:2043–2050.

8. Ferdinand KC. ASH Hypertension Community Outreach Program: taking actions to address "neglected" disease. *J Am Soc Hypertens* 2010;4(4):157–162.

9. Institute of Medicine. *Strategies to Reduce Sodium Intake in the United States.* Washington, DC: The National Academies Press, 2010.

10. Carter BL, Rogers M, Daly J, Zheng S, James PA. The potency of team-based care interventions for hypertension: a meta-analysis. *Arch Intern Med* 2009;169:1748–1755.

Appendix

Table A1 Classification and Management of Blood Pressure for Adults*

BP Classification	SBP mm Hg	DBP mm Hg	Lifestyle modifications	Initial Drug Therapy — Without Compelling Indication	Initial Drug Therapy — With Compelling Indications (See Table A3)
Normal	<120	and <80	Encourage	No antihypertensive drug indicated.	Drug(s) for compelling indications.[‡]
Prehypertension	120–139	or 80–89	Yes		
Stage 1 Hypertension	140–159	or 90–99	Yes	Thiazide-type diuretics for most. May consider ACEI, ARB, BB, CCB, or ombination.	Drug(s) for the compelling indications.[‡] Other antihypertensive drugs (diuretics, ACEI, ARB, BB, CCB) as needed.
Stage 2 Hypertension	≥160	or ≥100	Yes	Two-drug combination for most[†] (usually thiazidetype diuretic and ACEI or RB or BB or CCB).	

DBP, diastolic blood pressure; SBP, systolic blood pressure.

Drug abbreviations: ACEI, angiotensin converting enzyme inhibitor; ARB, angiotensin receptor blocker; BB, beta-blocker; CCB, calcium channel blocker.

* Treatment determined by highest BP category.

[†] Initial combined therapy should be used cautiously in those at risk for orthostatic hypotension.

[‡] Treat patients with chronic kidney disease or diabetes to BP goal of <130/80 mm Hg.

From the Seventh Report of the Joint National Committee on Prevention, Detection, Evaluation, and Treatment of High Blood Pressure. National Heart, Lung, and Blood Institute, National Institutes of Health, U.S. Department of Health and Human Services, December 2003.

Table A2 Lifestyle Modifications to Manage Hypertension*†

Modification	Recommendation	Approximate SBP Reduction (Range)
Weight reduction	Maintain normal body weight (body mass index 18.5–24.9 kg/m²).	5–20 mm Hg/10 kg weight loss[23,24]
Adopt DASH eating plan	Consume a diet rich in fruits, vegetables, and lowfat dairy products with a reduced content of saturated and total fat.	8–14 mm Hg[25,26]
Dietary sodium reduction	Reduce dietary sodium intake to no more than 100 mmol per day (2.4 g sodium or 6 g sodium chloride).	2–8 mm Hg[25–27]
Physical activity	Engage in regular aerobic physical activity such as brisk walking (at least 30 min per day, most days of the week).	4–9 mm Hg[28,29]
Moderation of alcohol consumption	Limit consumption to no more than consumption 2 drinks (1 oz or 30 mL ethanol; e.g., 24 oz beer, 10 oz wine, or 3 oz 80-proof whiskey) per day in most men and to no more than 1 drink per day in women and lighter weight persons.	2–4 mm Hg[30]

DASH, Dietary Approaches to Stop Hypertension.

* For overall cardiovascular risk reduction, stop smoking.

† The effects of implementing these modifications are dose and time dependent, and could be greater for some individuals.

From the Seventh Report of the Joint National Committee on Prevention, Detection, Evaluation, and Treatment of High Blood Pressure. National Heart, Lung, and Blood Institute, National Institutes of Health, U.S. Department of Health and Human Services, December 2003.

Table A3 Clinical trial and guideline basis for compelling indications for individual drug classes

Compelling Indication*	Diuretic	BB	ACEI	ARB	CCB	Aldo ANT	Clinical Trial Basis‡
Heart failure	•	•	•	•		•	ACC/AHA Heart Failure Guideline,[40] MERIT-HF,[41] COPERNICUS,[42] CIBIS,[43] SOLVD,[44] AIRE,[45] TRACE,[46] ValHEFT,[47] RALES[48]
Postmyocardial infarction		•	•			•	ACC/AHA Post-MI Guideline,[49] BHAT,[50] SAVE,[51] Capricorn,[52] EPHESUS[53]
High coronary disease risk	•	•	•		•		ALLHAT,[33] HOPE,[34] ANBP2,[36] LIFE,[32] CONVINCE[31]
Diabetes	•	•	•	•	•		NKF-ADA Guideline,[21,22] UKPDS,[54] ALLHAT[33]
Chronic kidney disease			•	•			NFK Guideline,[22] Captopril Trial,[55] RENAAL,[56] IDNT,[57] REIN,[58] AASK[59]
Recurrent stroke prevention	•		•				PROGRESS[35]

The top of the table reads: **Recommended Drugs†**

* Compelling indications for antihypertensive drugs are based on benefits from outcome studies or existing clinical guidelines; the compelling indication is managed in parallel with the BP.

† Drug abbreviations: ACEI, angiotensin converting enzyme inhibitor; ARB, angiotensin receptor blocker; Aldo ANT, aldosterone antagonist; BB, beta-blocker; CCB, calcium channel blocker.

‡ Conditions for which clinical trials demonstrate benefit of specific classes of antihypertensive drugs.

From the Seventh Report of the Joint National Committee on Prevention, Detection, Evaluation, and Treatment of High Blood Pressure. National Heart, Lung, and Blood Institute, National Institutes of Health, U.S. Department of Health and Human Services, December 2003.

Index

A

ACCORD BP (Action to
Control Cardiovascular
Risk in Diabetes Blood
Pressure) trial, 50, 66, 76,
128–129
Acebutolol, avoidance of, 56
ACE inhibitors. See
angiotensin-converting
enzyme inhibitors
Action to Control
Cardiovascular Risk in
Diabetes-Memory in
Diabetes (ACCORD-
MIND), 86
ADHERE database, 60
Adolescents. See Children
and adolescents
Aerobic exercise
recommendations, 40t,
41, 67, 164t
African Americans
DASH diet success, 147
HTN characteristics, 47
HTN epidemiology,
101–102
ischemic heart disease
(case study), 55
salt sensitivity, 126
treatment strategies, 102
AIRE (Acute Infarction
Ramipril Efficacy) study, 62
Aldosterone receptor
antagonists, 49. See
also Eplerenone;
Spironolactone
Aliskiren, 45, 49
ALLHAT (Antihypertensive
and Lipid-Lowering
Treatment to Prevent
Heart Attack Trial), 46,
49, 57
Alpha-beta-blockers, 113. See
also Labetalol
Alpha-blockers, 11, 49, 68.
See also Doxazosin
Alzheimer's disease (AD).
See Cerebrovascular
disease/cognitive function
Ambulatory BP
measurements
benefits/limitations, 19–20
devices, 20
special clinical situations,
20, 22
technique, 20

American College of Obstetricians and Gynecologists
(ACOG), 106
American Diabetes
Association (ADA), 50, 67
American Heart Association
monitor cuff size
recommendation,
16, 17t
American Indians, 100
Amiloride, 49
Amlodipine. See also
CAMELOT study
ACE inhibitor comparison,
47
in combination therapy, 48
diuretic therapy
comparison, 46, 48, 68
enalapril comparison, 47
for ischemic heart disease,
57–58
for PAD, 138
Amturinide
(hydrochlorothiazide), 49
Anemia, with heart failure,
61–63
Angiotensin-converting
enzyme inhibitors
(ACE-Is), 11, 34. See
also Captopril; Enalapril;
HOPE trial; Lisinopril;
Perindopril; Ramipril;
Trandolapril; Verapamil
amlodipine comparison, 47
ARBs compared with,
67–68
chlorthalidone comparison,
49
chronic HTN in pregnancy
contraindication, 48
in chronic kidney disease
patients, 50, 74, 78
data recommending use
of, 42
for diabetic hypertension,
67
for diabetic patients, 50
DRI comparison, 43–45
effectiveness in
microalbuminuria,
129–130
for heart failure patients, 62
for ischemic heart disease,
57
for metabolic syndrome,
129–130
thiazide diuretics with, 57

Angiotensin II receptor
blockers (ARBs), 11, 34.
See also Losartan
absence of cough side
effect, 45–46
ACE inhibitors compared
with, 67–68
chronic HTN in pregancy
contraindication, 115
for chronic kidney disease,
50, 74, 78
data recommending use
of, 42
diabetes risk reductions
from, 43
for diabetic hypertension,
67
for diabetic patients, 50
diuretics comparison, for
the elderly, 42
DRI comparison, 43–45
effectiveness in
microalbuminuria, 125
for heart failure patients, 62
for ischemic heart disease,
57
for metabolic syndrome,
130
thiazide diuretics with, 57
Antidepressant medications,
24t
Aortic aneurysm, 55
ARBS. See angiotensin II
receptor blockers
Asian/Pacific Islander
Americans (APIAs),
100–101
Aspirin, low-dose therapy, 111
Assessment and Follow-Up
(SHEAF) study, 19
Association of Advancement
of Medical Instrumentation
(AAMI), 19
Atenolol, 56
Atherosclerosis, 34, 47, 66,
83.85, 126, 135–136
Atherosclerosis Risk in
Communities (ARIC)
study, 83
Atorvastatin, 135
Avoiding Cardiovascular
Events through
Combination Therapy
in Patients Living
with Systolic HTN
(ACCOMPLISH) study,
47, 48, 68

167

B

Behavioral Risk Factor Surveillance System (BRFSS), 100
Benazepril, 48
Bergamo Nephrologic Diabetes Complications Trial (BENEDICT) study, 129–130
Beta-blockers, 11, 34, 47–48, 114t. See also Acebutolol; Atenolol; Bisoprolol; Carvedilol; Metoprolol succinate; Pindolol
actions of, 56
with CCBs, 56–57
for coronary artery disease, 50
for heart failure, 62
for ischemic heart disease, 56
with minoxidil, 48
for myocardial infarction, 50
for PAD, 138
with thiazide diuretics, 50
Bezafibrate Infarction Prevention Trial, 74
Bisoprolol, 56
Body mass index (BMI), 23, 60–61, 65, 127, 143, 146t
Boston Collaborative Drug Surveillance Program, 87
British Hypertension Society (BHS), 19

C

Calcium channel blockers (CCBs), 11. See also Amlodipine; Diltiazem; Verapamil
with beta-blockers, 56–57
for diabetic HTN, 68
diuretic therapy vs., 46
for ischemic heart disease, 56–57
monotherapy/combinations, 47
RAAS blockers vs., 47
Calcium supplementation, in preeclampsia, 111
CAMELOT (Comparison of Amlodipine vs. Enalapril to Limit Occurrences of Thrombosis) study, 47, 55
Candesartan, 62, 151, 154
Candesartan in Heart Failure Assessment of Reduction in Morbidity and Mortality (CHARM) trial, 62
Captopril, 93, 129
Cardiovascular disease (CVD)
ACE inhibitor treatment recommendation, 42, 43

beta blockers for, 47–48
lab tests for assessment, 32
markers for, 7–8, 8f, 11
medical history in diagnosis, 22–23
mortality risks/preventive measures, 11–12
predictive factors, 9–10
risk factors, 1, 2–4, 6–7
Cardiovascular Health Study, 9
Carotid artery disease, 55
Carvedilol, 56
Central adrenergic inhibitors, 113. See also Methyldopa
Cerebrovascular disease/cognitive function, 83–87
comorbidities
diabetes mellitus, 84–86
dyslipidemia, 86–87
HTN relationship with, 83–84
risk factors, 22, 76
studies of, 84
CHARM (Candesartan in Heart Failure Assessment of Reduction in Morbidity and Mortality) trial, 62
CHD (coronary heart disease)
active vs. placebo treatment, 11
deaths from, 4, 5f
HTN compared with, 6
PAD as increased risk for, 135–138
pulse pressure (PP) association, 9–10
risk factors, 3–9, 8f
Chicago Heart Association Detection Project in Industry, 9
Children and adolescents
causes of HTN
essential HTN, 119–120
secondary HTN, 119, 120t
childhood HTN definition, 117–118
evaluation of HTN, 120–121
measurement of BP, 118–119
treatment strategies, 121
Chlorthalidone, 49, 68, 155
Chronic HTN
causes in children, 119
metabolic syndrome complication, 124
outpatient treatment success, 93
in pregnancy, 105–106, 107–108, 112, 113–114
drug treatments, 114t
new-onset vs. chronic, 111
with superimposed preeclampsia, 108
risk factors, 83

Chronic kidney disease
Chronic kidney disease (CKD). See also End-stage renal disease
clinical trials related to, 165t
CV endpoints in individuals with, 74
glomerular HTN, 73–74
HTN/insulin resistance with, 65
and hypertension, 71
implications in heart failure, 74
management of HTN and, 77–78
mortality rates, 76f
predictive factors, 66
preservation of renal function, 71–72
stroke prevention implications, 74, 76
therapeutic scenarios, 50
Clevidipine, 96
Clonidine, 49, 96, 151, 154–155
Cognitive function. See Cerebrovascular disease/cognitive function
Columbia Aging Project, 85
Community programs, 157–161
Comorbidities management
cerebrovascular disease, cognitive function, 83–87
chronic kidney disease, 71–78
diabetic hypertension, 65–68
heart failure, 59–63
ischemic heart disease, 55–58
Congenital adrenal hyperplasia, 24t, 26
Coronary artery disease (CAD). See also EUROPA study
AHA BP recommendations, 55
amlodipine treatment, 47
BP target recommendations, 55–56
with heart failure, 59–60
therapeutic scenarios, 50
Corticosteroids, 23, 24t, 120t, 153t
Cuff/bladder (of BP monitor)
deflation phase, 20
inflation pressure recommendations, 17
placement recommendations, 16, 20
size recommendations, 17t

Cushing syndrome, 24t, 26, 32, 36t, 108
Cyclosporine, 24t, 153t

D

DASH (Dietary Approaches to Stop Hypertension) dietary plan
BP-lowering success, 31–32, 39, 40t, 67, 164t
exercise in addition to, 157
LDL-lowering success, 128
SBP-lowering success, 147
DBP (diastolic blood pressure)
age-related increases, 2
benefits of lowering, 10
chronic HTN and, 107
creatine-related levels, 71
DASH dietary-related changes, 39
death-related data, 4, 15
excess lowering concerns, 55–56
heart failure risks, 74
Korotkoff sounds, 17
orthostatic hypotension and, 126
predictive value of, 8–10
pregnancy recommendations, 106
relation to CVD events, 12
stroke death risks, 6, 66
sudden escalating HTN and, 112
Decongestants (pseudoephedrine), 24t
Dementia. See Cerebrovascular disease/cognitive function
Detection, Evaluation, and Treatment of High BP (JNC), 7
Devices used for measuring BP
ambulatory measurements, 20
home measurements, 19
office measurements, 17
Diabetes mellitus. See also ACCORD BP trial; SOLVD trial; Type 2 diabetes mellitus
ACE inhibitors/ARBs and, 42–43
assessment factor, 22, 32, 33–34, 33t
BP control targets, 50
cerebrovascular disease risks, 84–86
clinical trials related to, 165t
epidemiology of HTN in, 123–124
with heart failure, 60
in HTN risk factor cluster, 6, 7f, 8f, 10, 29, 32
therapeutic scenarios, 50

Diabetic hypertension
benefits of HTN treatment, 66–67
case study, 68
complications, 66
treatment recommendations, 67–68
type 2 diabetes, HTN pathogenesis, 65–66
Diagnosing hypertension, 15–26. See also Laboratory procedures
ambulatory BP mesurements
benefits/limitations, 19–20
devices, 20
special clinical situations, 20, 22
technique, 20
home BP mesurements
benefits/limitations, 18
devices, 19
normal reading data, 22t
proposed algorithm, 21f
special clinical situations, 19
technique, 18–19
medical history, 22–23
monitor cuff size recommendation, 16, 17t
office BP mesurements
benefits/limitations, 16
devices, 17
error situations, 18
normal reading data, 22t
proposed algorithm, 21f
technique, 16–17
physical examination, 23, 25–26, 25t
Diastolic blood pressure (DBP)
CHD risks, 9
ischemic heart disease risks, 4
JNC guidelines, 7
lowering in CAD, concerns, 55–56
men-women comparison, 3–4
predictive value of, 7–8, 8f, 10
pulse pressure and, 1, 2
stroke death risks, 6
in sudden escalating HTN, 112
Diet. See also DASH dietary plan
lab testing, 30
strategies for reducing HTN, 31, 32, 39, 40t, 41
Digital preference in BP measurement, 16
Digit Symbol Substitution Test, 86

Dihydropyridine amlodipine, 47, 50, 57, 68
Diltiazem, 56, 143, 147
Direct alpha-2 agonists, 49. See also Clonidine
Direct renin inhibitor (DRI)
absence of cough side effect, 45–46
ARBs/ACE inhibitor comparison, 43–45
Diuretic therapy. See also Furosemide; Spironolactone; Thiazide diuretics
ARBs comparison, for the elderly, 42
choice/combinations, 46, 48
for heart failure, 62
for ischemic heart disease, 57
for obesity/metabolic syndrome, 129
Doxazosin, 49, 93
DREAM (Diabetes Reduction Assessment with Ramipril and Rosiglitazone Medication) trial, 67
Dyslipidemia, 22
childhood risks, 121
dementia association, 86
lipid-lowering therapy, 87, 130–131, 137
metabolic syndrome and, 123, 145
obesity association, 60
PAD risk factors, 136
protective cholesterol effect, 86
risk factor identification, 102
statin therapy, 65, 87, 131, 137

E

Education and Research Towards Health (EARTH) Study, 100
Elderly people
ARB vs. diuretic therapy, 42
Cardiovascular Health Study, 9
CVD risks, 12
home BP measurement, 19
lower extremity PAD, 135
treatment for, 12
Enalapril, 47, 55. See also CAMELOT study
Enalaprilat, 95–96
End-stage renal disease (ESRD), 66, 71, 74, 76, 102
Eplerenone, 49, 57
Esmolol, 96

Essential HTN
  in children and
    adolescents, 117,
    119–122
  in glomerular disease, 73
  in pregnancy, 107, 108
  treatment strategies, 42,
    43f, 46–49
EUROPA (European Trial
  on Reduction of Cardiac
  Events with Perindopril in
  Stable Coronary Artery
  Disease) study, 57

F

Fenoldopam, 93, 96
Framingham Heart Study,
  1–2, 6, 7f, 55, 60, 62, 83,
  85, 86, 100, 136, 143
Furosemide, 154

G

Genetic testing, 31, 32
Gestational HTN, 108
Glomerular HTN, 73–74
Gordon syndrome
  (pseudohypoaldo-
  steronism type II), 24t

H

Heart failure (HF)
  beta-blockers for, 47–48
  chronic kidney disease
    in, 74
  clinical trials related to, 165t
  comorbidities
    anemia, 61–63
    coronary artery disease,
      59–60
    diabetes mellitus, 60
    obesity, 60–61
    renal failure, 61
  diastolic HTN reduction
    and, 7
  global data, 59
  mortality data, 3
  risk factors, 4, 6
  thiazide superiority, 46
Heart Protection Study
  (HPS), 131, 137
HELLP (Hemolysis Elevated
  Liver enzymes, Low
  Platelets) syndrome,
  106, 110
Hemorrhagic stroke, 5–6,
  112
High Blood Pressure
  Education Program
  Working Group
  (NHBPEP), 106
Home BP mesurements
  benefits/limitations, 18
  devices, 19

normal reading data, 22t
proposed algorithm, 21f
special clinical situations,
  19
technique, 18–19
HOPE (Heart Outcomes
  Prevention) trial, 42,
  57, 138
Hydralazine, 48, 112t, 114t
Hydrochlorothiazide, 48, 49,
  65, 68, 114t, 135, 138, 143,
  151, 155
Hyperaldosteronism, 24tr
Hypertension control
  regimen adherence,
    143–148
  clinical outcomes
  costs of, 144
  improvement strategies,
    146t
  influencing factors, 145t
  types of non-adherence,
    144t
  resistant hypertension
  causes of, 152t
  contraindicated
    medications, 153t
  defined, 151–152
  evaluation, management,
    152–155
  treatment strategies,
    154t
Hypertension in the Very
  Elderly (HYVET) trials,
  84
Hypertension Optimal
  Treatment (HOT) trial,
  127
Hypertensive Old People
  in Edinburgh (HOPE)
  study, 84
Hypertensive retinopathy
  classification, 25t
Hypertensive urgencies,
  emergencies, 93–96
  case study, 93
  epidemiology of, 95
  outpatient treatment,
    93–94
  therapeutic goal, 95
  treatment options, 95–96
  types of, 94
Hyperthyroidism, 24t
Hypothyroidism, 24t
HYVET trial, 12

I

Insulin resistance. See also
  Obesity and metabolic
  syndrome
  CVD/CKD association,
    65
  described, 124–125
  diabetes association, 85
  heart failure and, 60
  lifestyle interventions, 128

metabolic syndrome
  component, 123, 124
  thiazide diuretic cautions,
    129
International Society on
  Hypertension in Blacks
  (ISHIB), 102
International Verapamil-
  Trandolapril (INVEST)
  study, 138
Inter-Tribal Heart Project,
  100
Irbesartan in
  Microalbuminuria (IRMA)
  II trial, 130
Ischemic heart disease
  management
  ACE inhibitors/ARBs, 57
  beta-blockers, 56
  calcium-channel
    blockers, 56–57
  diuretics, 57
  treatment, 57–58
Ischemic stroke, 5–6
Israel Ischemic Heart Disease
  study, 84

J

Joint National Committee
  (JNC) on Detection,
  Evaluation, and Treatment
  of High BP, 7, 127

K

Kidney Disease Outcomes
  Quality Initiative
  (KDOQI) guidelines,
  77–78

L

Labetalol, 95, 112t, 113, 114t
Laboratory procedures, 29–37
  recommended tests,
    35t–36t
  testing for causes, 33t
    diet, 30
    genes, 31
    renin-angiotensin-
      aldosterone system,
      30, 34
  test selection
    CVD risk factors, 32–34
    genetic/primary causes,
      32
    Na/K intake, 31–32
Left ventricular hypertrophy
  (LVH), 23, 25–26, 60,
  66, 101
Liddle syndrome, 24t
Lifestyle modifications, 163t,
  164t. See also DASH
  dietary plan
  assessment, 43f

community factors, 145*t*, 147, 160
dietary modifications, 30, 31–32, 39, 40*t*, 41
for HTN management
in chronic kidney disease, 78*t*
in obesity/metabolic syndrome, 128
in PAD, 137
in pregnancy, 115
in resistant HTN, 152
in type 2 diabetes, 67
JNC 7 recommendations, 56
smoking cessation, 41, 137, 147
sodium restriction strategy, 40*t*, 41, 41*f*
Lisinopril, 46, 93, 151
Loop diuretics, 154. *See also* Furosemide
Losartan, 42, 130
Losartan Intervention for Endpoint Introduction (LIFE) trial, 42, 130

M

Magnesium sulfate (MgSO₄) therapy, 112–113
Maine-Syracuse Longitudinal Study of Hypertension, 83
Medical history in diagnosing HTN, 22–23
Metabolic syndrome. *See also* Obesity and metabolic syndrome
ACE inhibitors for, 129–130
CKD/microalbuminuria complications, 66, 125
defined, 124, 124*it*
epidemiology of HTN in, 123–124
identification in children, 120
Metformin/glyburide, 65
Methyldopa, 113, 114*t*
Metoprolol succinate, 56
Mexican-Americans, 99–100, 101
Microalbuminuria
ACE inhibitor effectiveness, 125, 129–130
ARBs effectiveness, 125
IRMA II trial, 130
monitoring for
in diabetic patients, 50, 65–66, 68
in metabolic syndrome, 123, 124*t*, 125
risk factor assessment, 32, 33–34
Mineralocorticoid receptor antagonists, 49

Minorities
epidemiology, control rates
African Americans, 101–102
American Indians, 100
Asian/Pacific Islander Americans, 100–101
Mexican-Americans, 99–100
treatment options, 102
Minoxidil, 48
Modification of Diet in Renal Disease (MDRD) study, 71
Monoamine oxidase inhibitors, 24*t*
Mortality rates
CAD/chronic HF, 59, 74
CKD, 74
declining age-adjusted CV rates, 159
men, SBP vs. DBP, 8–9
PAD, 135, 137
Multi-Ethnic Study of Atherosclerosis (MESA), 100
Multiple Risk Factor Intervention Trial (MRFIT), 4, 8–9
Myocardial infarction (MI)
adjusted hazard ratios, 6, 9*f*
beta-blockers for, 47–48
ramipril prevention of, 42
risk factors, 3, 6
survival factors, 6
treatment impact, 10–11

N

Na/K dietary intake, assessment of, 31–32
Nateglinide, 67
Nateglinide and Valsartan in Impaired Glucose Tolerance Outcomes Research (NAVIGATOR), 67
National Health and Nutrition Examination Survey (NHANES), 99
National Heart, Lung, and Blood Institute Twin Study, 83
National High Blood Pressure Program (NHBPEP), 7
National Kidney Foundation (NKF), 50
Nicardipine, 95–96
Nifedipine, 112*t*, 114*t*
sublingual capsules, 94
Nitrates, for heart failure, 62
Nitroglycerin, 95
Nitroprusside, 94, 95–96, 112*t*
Nonpharmacologic treatment strategies, 39–42. *See also* DASH dietary plan; Lifestyle modifications
aerobic exercise, 41
limited successes from, 42

smoking cessation, 41
sodium reduction, 41, 41*f*
NSAIDs (nonsteroidal anti-inflammatory drugs), 24*t*

O

Obesity
dyslipidemia association, 60
with heart failure, 60–61
obesity-related HTN, 99
Obesity and metabolic syndrome, 123–131
clinical features, pathophysiology
insulin resistance, 124–125
microalbuminuria, 125
orthostatic hypotension, 126
salt sensitivity, volume expansion, 125–126
stimulation of RAAS, 126–127
systolic HTN, 126
management strategies
ACE inhibitors, 129–130
ARBs, 130
diuretics, 129
lifestyle interventions, 128
lipid lowering therapy, 130–131
Office BP mesurements
benefits/limitations, 16
devices, 17
error situations, 18
normal reading data, 22*t*
proposed algorithm, 21*f*
technique, 16–17
Ongoing Telmisartan Alone and in Combination with Ramipril Global Endpoints Trial (ONTARGET), 43, 48, 76

P

Paraganglioma, 24*t*
Perindopril, 57, 67
Peripheral artery disease (PAD), 55, 135–138
atherosclerosis implications, 136
beta-blockers masking of symptoms, 68
case study, 135
causes/risk factors, 136
elderly people/lower extremities, 135
treatment strategies, 137–138
underdiagnosis, 137

Pharmacologic treatment strategies, 42–49. *See also* individual drugs
beta-blockers, 47–48
calcium-channel blockers, 46
combination therapy, 46
diuretic therapy, 46–47
RAAS blockade, 42–46
resistant HTN agents
mineralocorticoid receptor antagonists, 49
potassium-sparing diuretics, 49
special scenarios
chronic kidney disease, 50
coronary artery disease, 50
diabetes, 50
vasodilating agents
alpha-blockers, 49
hydralazine, 48
minoxidil, 48
sympatholytics, 49
Pheochromocytoma, 24t, 30, 32
Physical examination, 23, 25–26, 25t
Physicians' Health Study (PHS), 72
Pindolol, 56
Potassium-sparing diuretics, 49. *See also* Amiloride
Preeclampsia, 106
case study, 105, 115–116
pathogenic mechanisms, 108–109
pathophysiology of, 109–111
prediction, prevention of, 111
remote prognosis, 115
severity judgment, 107t
superimposed, with chronic HTN, 108
Pregnancy, HTN
classifications. *See also* Preeclampsia
chronic HTN, 105–106, 107–108, 112, 113–114
drug treatments, 114t
new-onset vs. chronic, 111
with superimposed preeclampsia, 108
CV and volume changes, 105–106
eclampsia, 107
gestational HTN, 108
management of HTN
chronic HTN, 113, 114t, 115
sudden escalating HTN, 112–113, 112t

obstetric management, 115
remote prognosis, 115
Preterax and Diamicron Modified Release Controlled Evaluation (ADVANCE) study, 66–67
Primary glomerular disease, pathophysiology of systemic HTN, 73–74
Prospective Randomized Evaluation of the Vascular Effects of Norvasc Trial (PREVENT), 47
Prospective Studies Collaboration, 4
Pseudoephedrine, 24t
Pulse pressure (PP), 1
central arterial stiffness and, 2
CHD, HF, stroke association, 9–10
SBP/DBP and, 2

R

RALES (Randomized Aldosterone Evaluation Study), 62
Ramipril, 42–43, 48, 62, 67, 129, 138, 143. *See also* AIRE (Acute Infarction Ramipril Efficacy) study
Reduction of Atherothrombosis for Continued Health (REACH) registry, 135
Regimen adherence, 143–148
clinical outcomes
costs of, 144
improvement strategies, 146t
influencing factors, 145t
types of non-adherence, 144t
Renal artery stenosis, 30
Renal failure
with heart failure, 61
Renin-angiotensin-aldosterone system (RAAS), 30, 65
Renin-angiotensin-aldosterone system (RAAS) blockade, 42–46, 48
Resistant hypertension
case study, 151
causes of, 152t
contraindicated medications, 153t
defined, 151–152
evaluation, management, 152–155
treatment strategies, 49, 154t

Risk factors
absolute/relative risks, 2
attributable risks, 3
cardiovascular disease, 1, 2–4, 6–7
cerebrovascular disease/cognitive function, 22, 76
chronic HTN, 83
clustering of, 6–7
coronary heart disease, 3–9, 8f
diabetes mellitus, clusters, 6, 7f, 8f, 10, 29, 32
heart failure, 4, 6
microalbuminuria, 32, 33–34
myocardial infarction, 3, 6
PAD risk factors, in dyslipemia, 136
peripheral artery disease, 136
Rosiglitazone, 67

S

Salt sensitivity issues, 124–126
SBP (systolic blood pressure)
atherosclerosis and, 126
benefits of lowering, 10, 11–12
as goal of treatment, 11–12
kidney function relation to, 72
Korotkoff sounds, 17
obesity/metabolic syndrome and, 127
predictive importance of, 7, 9
pulse pressure and, 2
reading underestimation, 17
Scandinavian Simvastatin Survival Study (4S), 131
Scientific Statement (AHA) (2007), 55
Secondary HTN
causes of, 24t
in children and adolescents, 119, 120t, 122
CKD and, 71
in hypertensive urgencies, emergencies, 95
in pregnancy, 107, 115
Self-Measurement of Blood Pressure at Home in the Elderly, 19
Serotonin inhibitors, 24t
Simvastatin, 65, 131, 137
Smoking cessation, 41, 137, 147
Sodium nitroprusside, 94
Sodium restriction strategy, 40t, 41, 41f

SOLVD (Left Ventricular Dysfunctions) trial, 60, 61
Special populations
children and adolescents, 117–122
hypertensive urgencies, emergencies, 93–96
minorities, 99–102
obesity and metabolic syndrome, 123–131
peripheral arterial disease, 135–138
pregancy, 105–116
Spironolactone, 49, 57, 62, 155
Statin therapy, 65, 87, 131, 137. *See also* Atorvastatin; Simvastatin
Stroke
ARB vs. diuretic therapy, 42
clinical trials related to, 165t
HTN and, 3–6
implications of CKD in, 74, 76
ischemic/hemorrhagic, 5–6
thiazide superiority, 46
Strong Heart Study, 100
Study of Women's Health Across the Nation (SWAN), 101
Study on Cognition and Prognosis in the Elderly (SCOPE), 42, 84
Sympatholytics, 49
Systolic Blood Pressure Intervention Trial (SPRINT), 84
Systolic Hypertension in Elderly Prevention (SHEP), 84
Systolic Hypertension in Europe (Syst-Eur) study, 84

T

Tacrolimus, 24t
Tekamlo (aliskiren), 49
Telmisartan, 43, 48
Terminal digit bias, 16
Thiazide diuretics, 46–47, 48, 50, 114t. *See also* Hydrochlorothiazide
ACE inhibitors/ARBs with, 57
for CKD, 78
in combination therapy, 48, 50
for diabetic HTN, 68
low-dose tolerability, 46
for obesity/metabolic syndrome, 129
risks of, in insulin resistance, 129
stroke/HF superiority, 46
Torsemide, 93, 154
Trandolapril, 130, 138
Treatment of essential HTN, 39–50
in the elderly, 12
goal for SBP, 11–12
nonpharmacologic strategies, 39–42
pharmacologic strategies, 42–49
Tricyclic antidepressants (TCAs), 24t
Truncal obesity, 26
Type 3 diabetes, 85
Type 2 diabetes mellitus
ACCORD BP trial data, 50, 76
assessment for, 22
benefits of treating HTN in, 66–67
complications related to HTN in, 66
obesity/metabolic syndrome and, 123–125, 128–130
pathogenesis of HTN in, 65–66

U

UK Prospective Diabetes Study (UKPDS), 66, 127
Uppsala Longitudinal Study of Adult Men, 85

V

VA Cooperative Trial, 10
Valsartan, 67, 138
Valsartan Antihypertensive Long-term Use Evaluation (VALUE) trial, 138
Vascular cognitive impairment (VCI). *See* Cerebrovascular disease/cognitive function
Vasodilating agents
alpha-blockers, 49
hydralazine, 48
minoxidil, 48
sympatholytics, 49
Verapamil, 56, 93, 129

W

Weight loss strategy. *See also* DASH dietary plan
diabetic HTN recommendation, 67
for obesity/metabolic syndrome, 128
for resistant HTN, 152–153
SBP reduction recommendation, 40t, 164t
"White coat" hypertension, 16–20, 119, 152, 152t

in peripheral arterial disease, 135
treatment recommendations, 67–68, 129–130